Neonatal
Nurse Practitioner
Exam
Part 1 of 2

SECRETS

Study Guide
Your Key to Exam Success

NP Test Review for the
Nurse Practitioner Exam

Dear Future Exam Success Story:

First of all, **THANK YOU** for purchasing Mometrix study materials!

Second, congratulations! You are one of the few determined test-takers who are committed to doing whatever it takes to excel on your exam. **You have come to the right place.** We developed these study materials with one goal in mind: to deliver you the information you need in a format that's concise and easy to use.

In addition to optimizing your guide for the content of the test, we've outlined our recommended steps for breaking down the preparation process into small, attainable goals so you can make sure you stay on track.

We've also analyzed the entire test-taking process, identifying the most common pitfalls and showing how you can overcome them and be ready for any curveball the test throws you.

Standardized testing is one of the biggest obstacles on your road to success, which only increases the importance of doing well in the high-pressure, high-stakes environment of test day. Your results on this test could have a significant impact on your future, and this guide provides the information and practical advice to help you achieve your full potential on test day.

Your success is our success

We would love to hear from you! If you would like to share the story of your exam success or if you have any questions or comments in regard to our products, please contact us at **800-673-8175** or **support@mometrix.com**.

Thanks again for your business and we wish you continued success!

Sincerely,
The Mometrix Test Preparation Team

Need more help? Check out our flashcards at: http://MometrixFlashcards.com/NP

TABLE OF CONTENTS

Introduction

Thank you for purchasing this resource! You have made the choice to prepare yourself for a test that could have a huge impact on your future, and this guide is designed to help you be fully ready for test day. Obviously, it's important to have a solid understanding of the test material, but you also need to be prepared for the unique environment and stressors of the test, so that you can perform to the best of your abilities.

For this purpose, the first section that appears in this guide is the **Secret Keys**. We've devoted countless hours to meticulously researching what works and what doesn't, and we've boiled down our findings to the five most impactful steps you can take to improve your performance on the test. We start at the beginning with study planning and move through the preparation process, all the way to the testing strategies that will help you get the most out of what you know when you're finally sitting in front of the test.

We recommend that you start preparing for your test as far in advance as possible. However, if you've bought this guide as a last-minute study resource and only have a few days before your test, we recommend that you skip over the first two Secret Keys since they address a long-term study plan.

If you struggle with **test anxiety**, we strongly encourage you to check out our recommendations for how you can overcome it. Test anxiety is a formidable foe, but it can be beaten, and we want to make sure you have the tools you need to defeat it.

Secret Key #1 – Plan Big, Study Small

There's a lot riding on your performance. If you want to ace this test, you're going to need to keep your skills sharp and the material fresh in your mind. You need a plan that lets you review everything you need to know while still fitting in your schedule. We'll break this strategy down into three categories.

Information Organization

Start with the information you already have: the official test outline. From this, you can make a complete list of all the concepts you need to cover before the test. Organize these concepts into groups that can be studied together, and create a list of any related vocabulary you need to learn so you can brush up on any difficult terms. You'll want to keep this vocabulary list handy once you actually start studying since you may need to add to it along the way.

Time Management

Once you have your set of study concepts, decide how to spread them out over the time you have left before the test. Break your study plan into small, clear goals so you have a manageable task for each day and know exactly what you're doing. Then just focus on one small step at a time. When you manage your time this way, you don't need to spend hours at a time studying. Studying a small block of content for a short period each day helps you retain information better and avoid stressing over how much you have left to do. You can relax knowing that you have a plan to cover everything in time. In order for this strategy to be effective though, you have to start studying early and stick to your schedule. Avoid the exhaustion and futility that comes from last-minute cramming!

Study Environment

The environment you study in has a big impact on your learning. Studying in a coffee shop, while probably more enjoyable, is not likely to be as fruitful as studying in a quiet room. It's important to keep distractions to a minimum. You're only planning to study for a short block of time, so make the most of it. Don't pause to check your phone or get up to find a snack. It's also important to **avoid multitasking**. Research has consistently shown that multitasking will make your studying dramatically less effective. Your study area should also be comfortable and well-lit so you don't have the distraction of straining your eyes or sitting on an uncomfortable chair.

The time of day you study is also important. You want to be rested and alert. Don't wait until just before bedtime. Study when you'll be most likely to comprehend and remember. Even better, if you know what time of day your test will be, set that time aside for study. That way your brain will be used to working on that subject at that specific time and you'll have a better chance of recalling information.

Finally, it can be helpful to team up with others who are studying for the same test. Your actual studying should be done in as isolated an environment as possible, but the work of organizing the information and setting up the study plan can be divided up. In between study sessions, you can discuss with your teammates the concepts that you're all studying and quiz each other on the details. Just be sure that your teammates are as serious about the test as you are. If you find that your study time is being replaced with social time, you might need to find a new team.

Secret Key #2 – Make Your Studying Count

You're devoting a lot of time and effort to preparing for this test, so you want to be absolutely certain it will pay off. This means doing more than just reading the content and hoping you can remember it on test day. It's important to make every minute of study count. There are two main areas you can focus on to make your studying count:

Retention

It doesn't matter how much time you study if you can't remember the material. You need to make sure you are retaining the concepts. To check your retention of the information you're learning, try recalling it at later times with minimal prompting. Try carrying around flashcards and glance at one or two from time to time or ask a friend who's also studying for the test to quiz you.

To enhance your retention, look for ways to put the information into practice so that you can apply it rather than simply recalling it. If you're using the information in practical ways, it will be much easier to remember. Similarly, it helps to solidify a concept in your mind if you're not only reading it to yourself but also explaining it to someone else. Ask a friend to let you teach them about a concept you're a little shaky on (or speak aloud to an imaginary audience if necessary). As you try to summarize, define, give examples, and answer your friend's questions, you'll understand the concepts better and they will stay with you longer. Finally, step back for a big picture view and ask yourself how each piece of information fits with the whole subject. When you link the different concepts together and see them working together as a whole, it's easier to remember the individual components.

Finally, practice showing your work on any multi-step problems, even if you're just studying. Writing out each step you take to solve a problem will help solidify the process in your mind, and you'll be more likely to remember it during the test.

Modality

Modality simply refers to the means or method by which you study. Choosing a study modality that fits your own individual learning style is crucial. No two people learn best in exactly the same way, so it's important to know your strengths and use them to your advantage.

For example, if you learn best by visualization, focus on visualizing a concept in your mind and draw an image or a diagram. Try color-coding your notes, illustrating them, or creating symbols that will trigger your mind to recall a learned concept. If you learn best by hearing or discussing information, find a study partner who learns the same way or read aloud to yourself. Think about how to put the information in your own words. Imagine that you are giving a lecture on the topic and record yourself so you can listen to it later.

For any learning style, flashcards can be helpful. Organize the information so you can take advantage of spare moments to review. Underline key words or phrases. Use different colors for different categories. Mnemonic devices (such as creating a short list in which every item starts with the same letter) can also help with retention. Find what works best for you and use it to store the information in your mind most effectively and easily.

Secret Key #3 – Practice the Right Way

Your success on test day depends not only on how many hours you put into preparing, but also on whether you prepared the right way. It's good to check along the way to see if your studying is paying off. One of the most effective ways to do this is by taking practice tests to evaluate your progress. Practice tests are useful because they show exactly where you need to improve. Every time you take a practice test, pay special attention to these three groups of questions:

- The questions you got wrong
- The questions you had to guess on, even if you guessed right
- The questions you found difficult or slow to work through

This will show you exactly what your weak areas are, and where you need to devote more study time. Ask yourself why each of these questions gave you trouble. Was it because you didn't understand the material? Was it because you didn't remember the vocabulary? Do you need more repetitions on this type of question to build speed and confidence? Dig into those questions and figure out how you can strengthen your weak areas as you go back to review the material.

Additionally, many practice tests have a section explaining the answer choices. It can be tempting to read the explanation and think that you now have a good understanding of the concept. However, an explanation likely only covers part of the question's broader context. Even if the explanation makes sense, **go back and investigate** every concept related to the question until you're positive you have a thorough understanding.

As you go along, keep in mind that the practice test is just that: practice. Memorizing these questions and answers will not be very helpful on the actual test because it is unlikely to have any of the same exact questions. If you only know the right answers to the sample questions, you won't be prepared for the real thing. **Study the concepts** until you understand them fully, and then you'll be able to answer any question that shows up on the test.

It's important to wait on the practice tests until you're ready. If you take a test on your first day of study, you may be overwhelmed by the amount of material covered and how much you need to learn. Work up to it gradually.

On test day, you'll need to be prepared for answering questions, managing your time, and using the test-taking strategies you've learned. It's a lot to balance, like a mental marathon that will have a big impact on your future. Like training for a marathon, you'll need to start slowly and work your way up. When test day arrives, you'll be ready.

Start with the strategies you've read in the first two Secret Keys—plan your course and study in the way that works best for you. If you have time, consider using multiple study resources to get different approaches to the same concepts. It can be helpful to see difficult concepts from more than one angle. Then find a good source for practice tests. Many times, the test website will suggest potential study resources or provide sample tests.

Practice Test Strategy

If you're able to find at least three practice tests, we recommend this strategy:

Untimed and Open-Book Practice

Take the first test with no time constraints and with your notes and study guide handy. Take your time and focus on applying the strategies you've learned.

Timed and Open-Book Practice

Take the second practice test open-book as well, but set a timer and practice pacing yourself to finish in time.

Timed and Closed-Book Practice

Take any other practice tests as if it were test day. Set a timer and put away your study materials. Sit at a table or desk in a quiet room, imagine yourself at the testing center, and answer questions as quickly and accurately as possible.

Keep repeating timed and closed-book tests on a regular basis until you run out of practice tests or it's time for the actual test. Your mind will be ready for the schedule and stress of test day, and you'll be able to focus on recalling the material you've learned.

Secret Key #4 – Pace Yourself

Once you're fully prepared for the material on the test, your biggest challenge on test day will be managing your time. Just knowing that the clock is ticking can make you panic even if you have plenty of time left. Work on pacing yourself so you can build confidence against the time constraints of the exam. Pacing is a difficult skill to master, especially in a high-pressure environment, so **practice is vital**.

Set time expectations for your pace based on how much time is available. For example, if a section has 60 questions and the time limit is 30 minutes, you know you have to average 30 seconds or less per question in order to answer them all. Although 30 seconds is the hard limit, set 25 seconds per question as your goal, so you reserve extra time to spend on harder questions. When you budget extra time for the harder questions, you no longer have any reason to stress when those questions take longer to answer.

Don't let this time expectation distract you from working through the test at a calm, steady pace, but keep it in mind so you don't spend too much time on any one question. Recognize that taking extra time on one question you don't understand may keep you from answering two that you do understand later in the test. If your time limit for a question is up and you're still not sure of the answer, mark it and move on, and come back to it later if the time and the test format allow. If the testing format doesn't allow you to return to earlier questions, just make an educated guess; then put it out of your mind and move on.

On the easier questions, be careful not to rush. It may seem wise to hurry through them so you have more time for the challenging ones, but it's not worth missing one if you know the concept and just didn't take the time to read the question fully. Work efficiently but make sure you understand the question and have looked at all of the answer choices, since more than one may seem right at first.

Even if you're paying attention to the time, you may find yourself a little behind at some point. You should speed up to get back on track, but do so wisely. Don't panic; just take a few seconds less on each question until you're caught up. Don't guess without thinking, but do look through the answer choices and eliminate any you know are wrong. If you can get down to two choices, it is often worthwhile to guess from those. Once you've chosen an answer, move on and don't dwell on any that you skipped or had to hurry through. If a question was taking too long, chances are it was one of the harder ones, so you weren't as likely to get it right anyway.

On the other hand, if you find yourself getting ahead of schedule, it may be beneficial to slow down a little. The more quickly you work, the more likely you are to make a careless mistake that will affect your score. You've budgeted time for each question, so don't be afraid to spend that time. Practice an efficient but careful pace to get the most out of the time you have.

Secret Key #5 – Have a Plan for Guessing

When you're taking the test, you may find yourself stuck on a question. Some of the answer choices seem better than others, but you don't see the one answer choice that is obviously correct. What do you do?

The scenario described above is very common, yet most test takers have not effectively prepared for it. Developing and practicing a plan for guessing may be one of the single most effective uses of your time as you get ready for the exam.

In developing your plan for guessing, there are three questions to address:

- When should you start the guessing process?
- How should you narrow down the choices?
- Which answer should you choose?

When to Start the Guessing Process

Unless your plan for guessing is to select C every time (which, despite its merits, is not what we recommend), you need to leave yourself enough time to apply your answer elimination strategies. Since you have a limited amount of time for each question, that means that if you're going to give yourself the best shot at guessing correctly, you have to decide quickly whether or not you will guess.

Of course, the best-case scenario is that you don't have to guess at all, so first, see if you can answer the question based on your knowledge of the subject and basic reasoning skills. Focus on the key words in the question and try to jog your memory of related topics. Give yourself a chance to bring the knowledge to mind, but once you realize that you don't have (or you can't access) the knowledge you need to answer the question, it's time to start the guessing process.

It's almost always better to start the guessing process too early than too late. It only takes a few seconds to remember something and answer the question from knowledge. Carefully eliminating wrong answer choices takes longer. Plus, going through the process of eliminating answer choices can actually help jog your memory.

Summary: Start the guessing process as soon as you decide that you can't answer the question based on your knowledge.

How to Narrow Down the Choices

The next chapter in this book (**Test-Taking Strategies**) includes a wide range of strategies for how to approach questions and how to look for answer choices to eliminate. You will definitely want to read those carefully, practice them, and figure out which ones work best for you. Here though, we're going to address a mindset rather than a particular strategy.

Your chances of guessing an answer correctly depend on how many options you are choosing from.

How many choices you have	How likely you are to guess correctly
5	20%
4	25%
3	33%
2	50%
1	100%

You can see from this chart just how valuable it is to be able to eliminate incorrect answers and make an educated guess, but there are two things that many test takers do that cause them to miss out on the benefits of guessing:

- Accidentally eliminating the correct answer
- Selecting an answer based on an impression

We'll look at the first one here, and the second one in the next section.

To avoid accidentally eliminating the correct answer, we recommend a thought exercise called **the $5 challenge**. In this challenge, you only eliminate an answer choice from contention if you are willing to bet $5 on it being wrong. Why $5? Five dollars is a small but not insignificant amount of money. It's an amount you could afford to lose but wouldn't want to throw away. And while losing $5 once might not hurt too much, doing it twenty times will set you back $100. In the same way, each small decision you make—eliminating a choice here, guessing on a question there—won't by itself impact your score very much, but when you put them all together, they can make a big difference. By holding each answer choice elimination decision to a higher standard, you can reduce the risk of accidentally eliminating the correct answer.

The $5 challenge can also be applied in a positive sense: If you are willing to bet $5 that an answer choice *is* correct, go ahead and mark it as correct.

Summary: Only eliminate an answer choice if you are willing to bet $5 that it is wrong.

Which Answer to Choose

You're taking the test. You've run into a hard question and decided you'll have to guess. You've eliminated all the answer choices you're willing to bet $5 on. Now you have to pick an answer. Why do we even need to talk about this? Why can't you just pick whichever one you feel like when the time comes?

The answer to these questions is that if you don't come into the test with a plan, you'll rely on your impression to select an answer choice, and if you do that, you risk falling into a trap. The test writers know that everyone who takes their test will be guessing on some of the questions, so they intentionally write wrong answer choices to seem plausible. You still have to pick an answer though, and if the wrong answer choices are designed to look right, how can you ever be sure that you're not falling for their trap? The best solution we've found to this dilemma is to take the decision out of your hands entirely. Here is the process we recommend:

Once you've eliminated any choices that you are confident (willing to bet $5) are wrong, select the first remaining choice as your answer.

Whether you choose to select the first remaining choice, the second, or the last, the important thing is that you use some preselected standard. Using this approach guarantees that you will not be enticed into selecting an answer choice that looks right, because you are not basing your decision on how the answer choices look.

This is not meant to make you question your knowledge. Instead, it is to help you recognize the difference between your knowledge and your impressions. There's a huge difference between thinking an answer is right because of what you know, and thinking an answer is right because it looks or sounds like it should be right.

Summary: To ensure that your selection is appropriately random, make a predetermined selection from among all answer choices you have not eliminated.

Test-Taking Strategies

This section contains a list of test-taking strategies that you may find helpful as you work through the test. By taking what you know and applying logical thought, you can maximize your chances of answering any question correctly!

It is very important to realize that every question is different and every person is different: no single strategy will work on every question, and no single strategy will work for every person. That's why we've included all of them here, so you can try them out and determine which ones work best for different types of questions and which ones work best for you.

Question Strategies

Read Carefully

Read the question and answer choices carefully. Don't miss the question because you misread the terms. You have plenty of time to read each question thoroughly and make sure you understand what is being asked. Yet a happy medium must be attained, so don't waste too much time. You must read carefully, but efficiently.

Contextual Clues

Look for contextual clues. If the question includes a word you are not familiar with, look at the immediate context for some indication of what the word might mean. Contextual clues can often give you all the information you need to decipher the meaning of an unfamiliar word. Even if you can't determine the meaning, you may be able to narrow down the possibilities enough to make a solid guess at the answer to the question.

Prefixes

If you're having trouble with a word in the question or answer choices, try dissecting it. Take advantage of every clue that the word might include. Prefixes and suffixes can be a huge help. Usually they allow you to determine a basic meaning. Pre- means before, post- means after, pro - is positive, de- is negative. From prefixes and suffixes, you can get an idea of the general meaning of the word and try to put it into context.

Hedge Words

Watch out for critical hedge words, such as *likely, may, can, sometimes, often, almost, mostly, usually, generally, rarely*, and *sometimes*. Question writers insert these hedge phrases to cover every possibility. Often an answer choice will be wrong simply because it leaves no room for exception. Be on guard for answer choices that have definitive words such as *exactly* and *always*.

Switchback Words

Stay alert for *switchbacks*. These are the words and phrases frequently used to alert you to shifts in thought. The most common switchback words are *but, although*, and *however*. Others include *nevertheless, on the other hand, even though, while, in spite of, despite, regardless of*. Switchback words are important to catch because they can change the direction of the question or an answer choice.

Face Value

When in doubt, use common sense. Accept the situation in the problem at face value. Don't read too much into it. These problems will not require you to make wild assumptions. If you have to go beyond creativity and warp time or space in order to have an answer choice fit the question, then you should move on and consider the other answer choices. These are normal problems rooted in reality. The applicable relationship or explanation may not be readily apparent, but it is there for you to figure out. Use your common sense to interpret anything that isn't clear.

Answer Choice Strategies

Answer Selection

The most thorough way to pick an answer choice is to identify and eliminate wrong answers until only one is left, then confirm it is the correct answer. Sometimes an answer choice may immediately seem right, but be careful. The test writers will usually put more than one reasonable answer choice on each question, so take a second to read all of them and make sure that the other choices are not equally obvious. As long as you have time left, it is better to read every answer choice than to pick the first one that looks right without checking the others.

Answer Choice Families

An answer choice family consists of two (in rare cases, three) answer choices that are very similar in construction and cannot all be true at the same time. If you see two answer choices that are direct opposites or parallels, one of them is usually the correct answer. For instance, if one answer choice says that quantity x increases and another either says that quantity x decreases (opposite) or says that quantity y increases (parallel), then those answer choices would fall into the same family. An answer choice that doesn't match the construction of the answer choice family is more likely to be incorrect. Most questions will not have answer choice families, but when they do appear, you should be prepared to recognize them.

Eliminate Answers

Eliminate answer choices as soon as you realize they are wrong, but make sure you consider all possibilities. If you are eliminating answer choices and realize that the last one you are left with is also wrong, don't panic. Start over and consider each choice again. There may be something you missed the first time that you will realize on the second pass.

Avoid Fact Traps

Don't be distracted by an answer choice that is factually true but doesn't answer the question. You are looking for the choice that answers the question. Stay focused on what the question is asking for so you don't accidentally pick an answer that is true but incorrect. Always go back to the question and make sure the answer choice you've selected actually answers the question and is not merely a true statement.

Extreme Statements

In general, you should avoid answers that put forth extreme actions as standard practice or proclaim controversial ideas as established fact. An answer choice that states the "process should be used in certain situations, if…" is much more likely to be correct than one that states the "process should be discontinued completely." The first is a calm rational statement and doesn't even make a definitive, uncompromising stance, using a hedge word *if* to provide wiggle room, whereas the second choice is a radical idea and far more extreme.

Benchmark

As you read through the answer choices and you come across one that seems to answer the question well, mentally select that answer choice. This is not your final answer, but it's the one that will help you evaluate the other answer choices. The one that you selected is your benchmark or standard for judging each of the other answer choices. Every other answer choice must be compared to your benchmark. That choice is correct until proven otherwise by another answer choice beating it. If you find a better answer, then that one becomes your new benchmark. Once you've decided that no other choice answers the question as well as your benchmark, you have your final answer.

Predict the Answer

Before you even start looking at the answer choices, it is often best to try to predict the answer. When you come up with the answer on your own, it is easier to avoid distractions and traps because you will know exactly what to look for. The right answer choice is unlikely to be word-for-word what you came up with, but it should be a close match. Even if you are confident that you have the right answer, you should still take the time to read each option before moving on.

General Strategies

Tough Questions

If you are stumped on a problem or it appears too hard or too difficult, don't waste time. Move on! Remember though, if you can quickly check for obviously incorrect answer choices, your chances of guessing correctly are greatly improved. Before you completely give up, at least try to knock out a couple of possible answers. Eliminate what you can and then guess at the remaining answer choices before moving on.

Check Your Work

Since you will probably not know every term listed and the answer to every question, it is important that you get credit for the ones that you do know. Don't miss any questions through careless mistakes. If at all possible, try to take a second to look back over your answer selection and make sure you've selected the correct answer choice and haven't made a costly careless mistake (such as marking an answer choice that you didn't mean to mark). This quick double check should more than pay for itself in caught mistakes for the time it costs.

Pace Yourself

It's easy to be overwhelmed when you're looking at a page full of questions; your mind is confused and full of random thoughts, and the clock is ticking down faster than you would like. Calm down and maintain the pace that you have set for yourself. Especially as you get down to the last few minutes of the test, don't let the small numbers on the clock make you panic. As long as you are on track by monitoring your pace, you are guaranteed to have time for each question.

Don't Rush

It is very easy to make errors when you are in a hurry. Maintaining a fast pace in answering questions is pointless if it makes you miss questions that you would have gotten right otherwise. Test writers like to include distracting information and wrong answers that seem right. Taking a little extra time to avoid careless mistakes can make all the difference in your test score. Find a pace that allows you to be confident in the answers that you select.

Keep Moving

Panicking will not help you pass the test, so do your best to stay calm and keep moving. Taking deep breaths and going through the answer elimination steps you practiced can help to break through a stress barrier and keep your pace.

Final Notes

The combination of a solid foundation of content knowledge and the confidence that comes from practicing your plan for applying that knowledge is the key to maximizing your performance on test day. As your foundation of content knowledge is built up and strengthened, you'll find that the strategies included in this chapter become more and more effective in helping you quickly sift through the distractions and traps of the test to isolate the correct answer.

Now it's time to move on to the test content chapters of this book, but be sure to keep your goal in mind. As you read, think about how you will be able to apply this information on the test. If you've already seen sample questions for the test and you have an idea of the question format and style, try to come up with questions of your own that you can answer based on what you're reading. This will give you valuable practice applying your knowledge in the same ways you can expect to on test day.

Good luck and good studying!

General Assessment

Maternal Assessment: Antepartum

Fetal Exposure

<u>Fetal Exposure to Pregnancy-Induced Hypertension</u>

Pregnancy-induced hypertension (also called pre-eclampsia or toxemia) is a disorder that develops in approximately 5% of all pregnancies. Its main features are elevated blood pressure and proteinuria that develop around 20 weeks of gestation. Initial treatment of pre-eclampsia is magnesium sulfate to prevent seizures in the mother. Severe cases may require the premature delivery of the infant to relieve the condition. The main detrimental effect on the fetus occurs because of longstanding hypertension that leads to utero-placental vascular insufficiency, which impairs the transfer of nutrients and oxygen to the fetus, resulting in intrauterine growth retardation (IUGR). Placental abruption also occurs more frequently. The IUGR is usually asymmetric (fetal head size is normal for gestational age). Infants who are born with IUGR and/or prematurity have increased morbidity and mortality.

<u>Fetal Exposure to Classes I-IV Cardiac Disease</u>

The **NY Heart association classifies heart disease** by the functional capacity, and the maternal classification affects the fetus:

> I. No cardiac insufficiency or activity limitations.
> II. Slight activity limitations with symptoms present with ordinary physical activity.
> III. Marked activity limitations with mild activity causing symptoms.
> IV. Inability to carry out physical activities without severe symptoms.

There is minimal danger to the fetus for mothers in class I or II but increased risk to both the mother and the fetus for classes III and IV. Most mediations cross the placenta and the degree of safety during pregnancy has not always been established although most common drugs (heparin, digitalis glycosides, antiarrhythmics, thiazide and loop diuretics) are not teratogenic. For classes III and IV, delivery may be facilitated by low forceps or vacuum assistance, and Caesarean may be done if mother or fetus is in danger. Labor and delivery are particularly dangerous to the fetus because of inadequate oxygen and blood supply, so continuous fetal monitoring is essential.

<u>Fetal Exposure to Cardiopulmonary Defects</u>

With improved techniques of surgical repair of **congenital heart defects,** many women survive to childbearing age. Common maternal defects include tetralogy of Fallot, ventricular and atrial septal defects, patent ductus arteriosus, and coarctation of aorta. If surgical correction was successful, there is no added fetal risk, but if the condition was not completely repaired or involves cyanosis, pregnancy can put the fetus at risk because of inadequate oxygen supply (and 2-4% risk that the child will inherit the condition).

- *Marfan's syndrome* poses severe risks to the mother with mortality rates of 25-50% because of possible rupture of the aorta—also putting the fetus at risk. Additionally, because this is an autosomal dominant disorder, there is a 50% chance an infant will inherit.
- *Mitral valve prolapse* usually does not pose a risk to the fetus. Severe maternal cardiopulmonary disorders can result in death of the mother and/or fetus. However, the most common fetal complications are premature labor/birth and small for gestational age.

- 15 -

Fetal Exposure to Diabetes Mellitus

Infants of diabetic mothers (IDM) suffer from increased morbidity and mortality. Glucose crosses the placenta, so when the mother has elevated blood glucose, the infant also has elevated blood glucose. Insulin does not cross the placenta. The pancreas of the fetus begins to produce insulin at about 20 weeks of gestation. Prior to the fetus producing insulin, the infant is exposed to elevated levels of glucose that restrict fetal growth. After the 20 weeks, the fetus responds to hyperglycemia with elevated production of insulin. The combination of elevated blood glucose and elevated insulin triggers rapid fetal growth, with increased fat and glycogen stores, hepatosplenomegaly, cardiomegaly, and increased head size. Sudden withdrawal from the consistent maternal source of glucose after birth, combined with the continued production of insulin by the newborn, result in hypoglycemia shortly after birth.

Fetal Exposure to Malnutrition

Maternal malnutrition can have a profound effect on the developing fetus. If malnutrition occurs during the stages of cell division, then cells may not divide properly, causing permanent damage. If malnutrition occurs when cells are enlarging, then correcting the nutritional deficit can reverse damage. Maternal weight gain must be adequate:

- Underweight: 28-40 lb.
- Normal weight: 25-35 lb.
- Overweight: 15-25 lb.
- Obese: 15 lb.

Mothers who are malnourished or underweight have increased perinatal losses and preterm births. Neonates often have lower Apgar score and low birth weight (<2500 g). Women with eating disorders are more likely to have infants that are small for gestational age. Vitamin and mineral deficiencies can result in a number of problems for the developing fetus:

- Thiamine: Congestive heart failure, stillbirths.
- Folic acid: Megaloblastic anemia, neural tube defects.
- Vitamin D and calcium: Skeletal defects.

Infants of obese and morbidly obese women are often macrosomic (large) and may suffer fetal distress, early neonatal death, meconium aspiration, shoulder dystocia, and/or complications from Caesarean birth.

Fetal Exposure Sickle Cell Anemia

Sickle cell disease is a recessive genetic disorder of chromosome 11, causing hemoglobin to be defective so that red blood cells (RBCs) are sickle-shaped and inflexible, resulting in their accumulating in small vessels and causing painful blockage. There are 5 variations of sickle cell disease, with sickle cell anemia the most severe. Pregnant women with sickle cell anemia are at risk for urinary and pulmonary infections, congestive heart failure, and acute renal failure, all of which can trigger a vaso-occlusive crises that puts the fetus at risk, with perinatal mortality rates of about 18%, caused by sickling in the placenta. Neonates are at increased risk for prematurity and intrauterine growth restriction. Maternal infections must be treated promptly to avoid dehydration and/or fever that can trigger sickling. Steps to shorten the second stage of labor (oxytocin, forceps, episiotomy) may be necessary to protect the fetus if sickling occurs during labor.

Fetal Exposure Iron-Deficiency Anemia

Iron-deficiency anemia is a common complication of pregnancy, as plasma volume expansion is not met by adequate increase in hemoglobin. Because women generally have no menses during pregnancy, they conserve about 200 mg daily, but women require an increase of 1000 mg of iron over that amount because of increased needs of the mother, placenta, and fetus, especially in the last half of pregnancy. When hemoglobin falls <11 g/dL, the mother is at increased risk of infection, pre-eclampsia, and postpartal hemorrhage with associated dangers to the fetus. If hemoglobin falls <6 g/dL, the mother may suffer cardiac failure, and the fetus is at high risk through increased rates of miscarriage and stillbirths, low birth rate, and neonatal death. Neonates are not deficient of iron at birth but have low stores and may develop iron-deficiency, so the infant should be monitored carefully.

Fetal Exposure Folic Acid Deficiency Anemia

Folate/Folic acid is necessary for synthesis of DNA and RNA and cell duplication. **Folic acid deficiency** causes megaloblastic anemia in which immature red blood cells enlarge rather than divide, resulting in fewer red blood cells. Because of the need for cell duplication during pregnancy, adequate folic acid is critical, especially because there is increased urinary excretion and fetal uptake. Women should receive 0.4mg folic acid daily and, for deficiency, 1mg folic acid and iron supplements (because folic acid deficiency is associated with iron deficiency anemia). Deficiency may be difficult to diagnose because folate levels fluctuate with diet. Women with inadequate folic acid intake often exhibit nausea, vomiting, lack of appetite and low hemoglobin. Folic acid deficiency is associated with neural tube defects, such as myelomeningocele, spina bifida, and anencephaly, in the fetus.

Fetal Exposure Rh Sensitivity

Rh (D) sensitivity may occur when a Rh-negative mother's blood contacts blood of a Rh-positive fetus, resulting in anti-D antibodies that can cross the placenta and attack the fetal Rh-positive red blood cells, resulting in hemolysis. This is primarily a problem during second or subsequent pregnancies. Sensitization can occur during abortion, abruptio placentae, amniocentesis, cesarean section, chorionic villus sampling, cordocentesis, delivery, ectopic pregnancy, and toxemia. In the fetus, hemolysis triggers increased RBC production (erythroblastosis fetalis), a form of anemia that left untreated results in severe/fatal edema (hydrops fetalis) that can cause congestive heart failure. Hyperbilirubinemia and jaundice occur from RBC destruction, leading to neurological impairment (kernicterus). Prenatal antibody screening (indirect Coombs' test) to identify sensitized women and development of RhIG (RhoGAM®) has markedly decreased incidence. Management of fetal hemolysis may include early delivery (≥32 weeks after confirmation of pulmonary maturity if possible), with risks associated with prematurity, and intrauterine transfusion, which can cause fetal distress, hematoma, maternal-fetal hemorrhage, and fetal death (10-20%).

Fetal Exposure ABO Compatibility

About 20-25% of pregnancies involve **ABO incompatibility**, usually with the mother type O and the fetus A or B. Anti-A and anti-B antibodies occur naturally when a woman is exposed to A and B antigens in foods or bacteria, so these antibodies can cross the placenta and result in hemolysis of fetal RBC; however, the antibodies are relatively large and do not enter the fetal circulation easily. If fetal blood leaks into maternal blood (a common occurrence), then smaller antibodies form and these can cross the placenta more easily. There is no difference in affect between the first pregnancy and subsequent pregnancies. There are rarely serious complications for the fetus although the neonate may develop hyperbilirubinemia, so the child should be observed carefully.

Only in severe cases of hemolysis (rare), does the child require exchange transfusions. Anemia may develop in the weeks after delivery because of increased rate of RBC breakdown, so the neonate should be monitored with blood counts.

CHEAP TORCHES

CHEAP TORCHES is the acronym used to recall common causes of congenital and neonatal infections. Many congenital infections are present for at least a month prior to birth and remain present at birth:

Chickenpox (varicella)
Hepatitis (B, C, & E)
Enterovirus (RNA viruses, including coxsackievirus, echovirus, and poliovirus)
AIDS (HIV)
Parvovirus (B 19)

Toxoplasmosis
Other (Group B streptococcus, Candida, Listeria, TB, lymphocytic choriomeningitis)
Rubella (measles)
Cytomegalovirus
Herpes simplex virus
Every other STD (Chlamydia, gonorrhea, Ureaplasma, papillomavirus
Syphilis

Exposure to these pathogens *in utero* may cause a miscarriage or congenital defect, especially if the exposure was during the first trimester.

Fetal Exposure Varicella

Varicella infection (chickenpox) in the mother can affect the fetus in different ways, depending upon the time of exposure. ***Congenital varicella syndrome*** is characterized by many abnormalities, including eye abnormalities (cataracts, microphthalmia, pendular nystagmus and retinal scarring), skin abnormalities (hypertrophy and cicatrix scarring), malformation of limbs, hypoplasia of digits, retarded growth, microcephalus, abnormalities of the brain and autonomic nervous system, developmental delay, and intellectual disability. Mortality rates are high ($\geq$50%) for those with severe defects:

- First trimester: 1% risk of congenital varicella syndrome.
- Weeks 23-20: 2% risk of congenital varicella syndrome.
- 5 days before delivery to 2 days after delivery: Neonate may develop congenital varicella (20-25%).

6-12 days after delivery: Neonate may contract congenital varicella but, if breast-feeding, the child may receive the mother's antibodies so the disease will be milder.

Fetal Exposure Hepatitis (B, C, & E)

Routine screening of all pregnant women and all newborns helps to identify those infected with **hepatitis B virus (HBV)**. Infants are routinely immunized at discharge from hospital, at 2 months and at 6 months of age. In the case of a premature infant, the immunization schedule is started when the infant weighs 2 kg or is 2 months old. If the mother is HBV positive, surface antigen treatment of that infant should include careful bathing (wearing gloves) to remove all maternal blood and body fluids. The infant should also receive an IM injection of the hepatitis B immunoglobulin within 12 hours of birth. This immunoglobulin treatment is up to 95% effective in preventing the development of the disease in the infant. **Hepatitis C** is rarely transmitted to the fetus and of those infected about 75% clear the infection by 2 years. **Hepatitis E** poses the greatest risk to the mother with a mortality of about 20% during pregnancy and increased risk of fetal complications and death.

Fetal Exposure to Tuberculosis

Tuberculosis (TB), infection with *Mycobacterium tuberculosis,* does not appear to worsen with pregnancy and responds to treatment, and risk of transmission to the fetus is low. However, the fetus may acquire the infection directly from the mother's blood or from swallowing amniotic fluid although most transmission occurs post-partum through maternal contact, so mothers with active disease should not have contact with a neonate until they are noninfectious. Fetal infection may cause death of the fetus, increased risk of miscarriage, or neonatal infection. If the mother's TB is untreated, the fetal death rate is 30-40%, so treating the mother during pregnancy is very important. Isoniazid (INH), rifampin, and ethambutol cross the placenta, but do not appear to be teratogenic, and the need for treatment outweighs risks. Streptomycin should be avoided as it may result in sensorineural deafness in the neonate. Mothers with inactive disease taking medications may breastfeed.

Fetal Exposure Enterovirus

Enteroviruses include coxsackievirus, echovirus, and poliovirus (essentially eradicated in the United States). Most enterovirus infections (90%) in adults are asymptomatic or non-specific febrile illness with flu-like symptoms. There is no consensus regarding neonatal infections, but most researchers believe they are not acquired transplacentally but that infection occurs perennially (during delivery) or after birth (≥ 2 weeks) from exposure to a mother with the virus or another infected infant. Neonates are at increased risk of developing sepsis-like conditions, such as aseptic meningitis, myocarditis, and hepatitis. It may be difficult to differentiate enterovirus infection from bacterial sepsis. Because of lack of immune response, neonates <10 days are at increased risk from non-polio enteroviruses. Neonates may be lethargic, feverish, and exhibit signs of hypoperfusion (mottled skin, delay in capillary refill time, and cyanosis) and jaundice. They often feed poorly and cry inconsolably.

Fetal Exposure AIDS/HIV

Most children infected with **AIDS/HIV** acquire the infection from their mothers (vertical transmission). The perinatal transmission rate is 30% in untreated HIV positive mothers, usually acquired during delivery. Neonates are usually asymptomatic but are at risk for prematurity, low birth weight, and small for gestational age (SVA). Infants may show failure to thrive, hepatomegaly, interstitial lymphocytic pneumonia, recurrent infections, and CNS abnormalities. Optimal treatment reduces the perinatal transmission rate to as low as 1-2%:

- Antiviral therapy during the pregnancy: A reduced viral load in the mother lessens the likelihood of prenatal transmission.
- Elective caesarian section before the amniotic membranes rupture. Emergency caesarian, rupture of membranes longer than 4 hours, and the need for an episiotomy all increase the likelihood of infection during delivery.
- Antiviral medications for the neonate for the first 6 weeks of life. The first dose should be given within the first 6-12 hours after delivery.
- Avoiding breastfeeding: The risk of HIV transmission with breastfeeding is 0.7% per month of breastfeeding.

Fetal Exposure Parvovirus (B19)

Parvovirus B19 is a DNA virus that is very common and causes fever and malaise and depression of progenitor cells in the bone marrow with a drop in reticulocyte count that can lead to anemia in those with preexisting low blood count. Most people are asymptomatic although they can develop generalized rash and arthralgia/arthritis. Most mothers (≥50%) are seropositive with parvovirus before pregnancy, and can become reinfected during pregnancy. Most infections do not adversely affect the fetus, but about 1-2% of maternal infections may cause spontaneous abortion or nonimmune hydrops fetalis. Hydrops fetalis is characterized by marked anemia, cardiac failure, and extramedullary hematopoiesis. A Parvovirus congenital infection syndrome may also occur with rash, anemia, and enlargement of the heart and liver.

Fetal Exposure Toxoplasmosis

Toxoplasmosis, caused by a protozoal infection with *Toxoplasma gondii,* is a common disease. About 38% of pregnant women have antibodies from previous infection, but about 1 in 1000 pregnant women become infected during pregnancy, primarily from eating undercooked meat, drinking unpasteurized goat's milk, or contacting infected cat feces, putting the fetus at risk. Risk to the fetus is greatest if the disease occurs during the first trimester, often causing severe fetal abnormalities, such as microcephaly and hydrocephalus, or miscarriage. However, risk of fetal transmission is greatest during the 3rd trimester although 70% are born without indications of infection. Mild infection may be manifest by retinochoroiditis at birth (with other symptoms delayed). Severe infection may result in convulsions and coma from CNS abnormalities, and the child may die in the neonatal period. Children who survive with severe infection may suffer blindness, deafness, and marked intellectual disability. If diagnosis of fetal infection is made during pregnancy, the mother should be treated aggressively.

Fetal Exposure Group B Streptococcus (GBS)

Group B *Streptococcus* is the most common neonatal bacterial infection. Many women are asymptomatic carriers. Screening of all pregnant women around 36 weeks of gestation followed by antibiotic treatment of the mother during labor can prevent neonatal infection. A mother needs at least 4 hours' worth of antibiotic treatment for the infant to benefit. If an infant is born and the mother has not received the recommended treatment, the infant will often be treated with IV ampicillin and gentamicin for 10 to 14 days. If treatment is ineffective or impossible, the infant with a GBS infection that manifests in the first 24 hours after birth may develop pneumonia and/or meningitis, respiratory distress, floppiness, poor feeding, tachycardia, shock and seizures. An infant may be asymptomatic at birth but have late-onset infection occurring at around 7 to 10 days old. Late-onset infections (usually meningitis) are generally more serious than earlier onset, and survivors often have serious damage, such as intellectual disability, quadriplegia, blindness, deafness, uncontrollable seizures, and hydrocephalus.

Fetal Exposure Rubella

Women should always be vaccinated for **rubella** before becoming pregnant as exposure to the virus has devastating effects on the newborn. The mother may not experience any symptoms of the disease or only mild symptoms like mild respiratory problems or rash. If the rubella exposure is during the first 4 to 5 months of pregnancy, the consequences for the infant are greater. Infants exposed to this virus *in utero* can develop a set of symptoms known as congenital rubella syndrome. This syndrome includes all or some of the following signs and symptoms:

- Intrauterine growth retardation (IUGR).
- Deafness.
- Cataracts.

- Jaundice.
- Purpura.
- Hepatosplenomegaly.
- Microcephaly.
- Chronic encephalitis.
- Cardiac defects.

Fetal Exposure Cytomegalovirus

Cytomegalovirus, a member of the herpes simplex virus group, can cause asymptomatic infection in women. Over 50% of women are seropositive and may have chronic infections that persist for years. Cytomegalovirus is the most common intrauterine viral infection. Cytomegalovirus can be transmitted placentally or cervically during delivery (infecting ≥2.5% of neonates) and can put the fetus at high risk with death rates of 20-30% among infants born with symptoms. About 90% of survivors have neurological disorders, such as microcephaly, hydrocephalus, cerebral palsy, and/or intellectual disability. In less severe infections, symptoms (intellectual disability, hearing deficits, learning disabilities) may be delayed. Commonly, the neonate is small for gestational age (SVA). The brain and liver are commonly affected, but all organs can be infected. Multiple blood abnormalities can occur: anemia, hyperbilirubinemia, thrombocytopenia, and hepatosplenomegaly.

Fetal Exposure Herpes Simplex Virus

Most pregnant women infected with **herpes simplex virus** (HSV) are asymptomatic and unaware of infection. Most vertical transmissions occur when the neonate travels through a colonized birth canal. The risk of transmitting HSV during the birth process varies greatly, depending if the infection is a new infection (primary) or a secondary outbreak. The transmission rate from women with a primary HSV infection is approximately 50%, while the transmission rate is 1-2% if the infection is a recurrence of HSV. Signs of a neonatal infection with HSV include:

- Skin, eye, and mucous membrane blistering at 10—12 days of life.
- Disseminated disease may spread to multiple organs, leading to pneumonitis, hepatitis, and intravascular coagulation.
- Encephalitis may be the only presentation, with signs of lethargy, irritability, poor feeding, and seizures.

A mother with active herpes should deliver by cesarean section within 4-6 hours after membranes rupture. An infant is inadvertently exposed to an active lesion should be treated with acyclovir.

Fetal Exposure Chlamydia

Chlamydia is the most common sexually transmitted disease in the United States and can be passed on at the time of birth if the infant is delivered vaginally and comes into contact with contaminated vaginal secretions. The organism responsible for this infection is *Chlamydia trachomatis*. Because the mother infected with this organism is usually asymptomatic, preventative care for the newborn is essential. The usual infection site for the newborn is the eyes in the form of conjunctivitis. States now require all newborns be given a prophylactic dose of either erythromycin or tetracycline ointment in the eyes at birth to prevent this infection. While the antibiotic ointment stops the eye infection, a few infants exposed to the pathogen will develop pneumonitis and/or ear infection.

Fetal Exposure Syphilis

An infant can be exposed to the **syphilis** organism, *Treponema pallidum*, during gestation and become infected *in utero* starting with the 10th-15th week of gestation. Many infected fetuses abort spontaneously or are stillborn. The infant born infected with syphilis can be asymptomatic at birth or can have a full multi-system infection. An infant who is symptomatic may have non-viral hepatitis with jaundice, hepatosplenomegaly, pseudoparalysis, pneumonitis, bone marrow failure, myocarditis, meningitis, anemia, edema associated with nephritic syndrome, and a rash on the palms of the hands and soles of the feet.   Other symptoms, such as interstitial keratitis and dental and facial abnormalities may occur as the child develops. Treatment involves an aggressive regimen of penicillin administration with frequent follow-up until blood tests are negative.

Fetal Exposure Alcohol

Fetal alcohol syndrome (FAS) is a syndrome of birth defects that develop as the result of maternal ingestion of alcohol. Despite campaigns to inform the public, women continue to drink during pregnancy, but no safe amount of alcohol ingestion has been determined. FAS includes:

- *Facial abnormalities*: Hypoplastic (underdeveloped) maxilla, micrognathia (undersized jaw), hypoplastic philtrum (groove beneath the nose), short palpebral fissures (eye slits between upper and lower lids).
- *Neurological deficits*: May include microcephaly, intellectual disability, and motor delay, hearing deficits. Learning disorders may include problems with visual-spatial and verbal learning, attention disorders, delayed reaction times.
- *Growth retardation:* Prenatal growth deficit persists with slow growth after birth.
- *Behavioral problems:* Irritability and hyperactivity. Poor judgment in behavior may relate to deficit in executive functions.
- Indication of brain damage without the associated physical abnormalities is referred to as *alcohol-related neurodevelopmental disorder (ARND).*

Fetal Exposure Tobacco/Nicotine

Tobacco smoke contains many substances known to be detrimental to a person's health. When a pregnant woman smokes, her fetus is exposed to carbon monoxide, nicotine, and hydrogen cyanide that all cross the placenta. Carbon monoxide displaces oxygen from hemoglobin, resulting in decreased oxygen delivery to the fetus. Exposure increases risk of miscarriage and perinatal death. Infants exposed *in utero* to tobacco may have the following problems:

- Decreased length, weight, and head circumference.
- Increased rates of congenital birth defects, such as cleft palate or lip, limb reduction defects, and urinary tract anomalies.
- Increased incidence of placenta previa, placental abruption, and preterm birth.

If smoking continues after delivery, these further detrimental effects may occur:

- Sudden infant death syndrome.
- Increased infant respiratory tract infections and childhood asthma.
- Behavioral problems in later childhood.

Fetal Exposure Marijuana, Phencyclidine, and MDMA

Marijuana, phencyclidine (PCP), and methylenedioxymethamphetamine (MDMA or ecstasy) are popular and "club" drugs that may be used by some women during pregnancy:

- **Marijuana**: This is often used along with alcohol and tobacco, so effects are difficult to assess, but there do not appear to be teratogenic effects; however, some studies report exposure can result in fine tremors, irritability, and prolonged startle response for the first 12 months after birth.
- **PCP**: One of the biggest problems with PCP is that mothers may have an overdose or psychotic response that can result in hypertension, hyperthermia, and coma, compromising the fetus.
- **MDMA**: Ecstasy is a popular club drug that is frequently used by teenagers and young adults. There is no clear evidence regarding effects on the fetus although some research suggests it may cause long-term impairments in learning.

Fetal Exposure Amphetamines

Amphetamines are a class of drugs that cause CNS stimulation. The most commonly abused amphetamine is methamphetamine. Maternal use of these substances causes hypertension and tachycardia, which can cause miscarriage, abruptio placentae, and premature delivery. Vasoconstriction affects placental vessels, decreasing circulation, nutrition, and oxygen to the fetus. Methamphetamines can cross the placental barrier and cause fetal hypertension and prenatal strokes and damage to the heart and other organs. The neonate is commonly small for gestational age, often ≥ 5 pounds, full term but ≥10 percentile for weight, with shortened length and smaller head circumference. The neonate in withdrawal from maternal amphetamine use will suffer abnormal sleep patterns, often characterized by lethargy and excessive sleeping during the first few weeks, poor feeding, tremors, diaphoresis, miosis, frantic fist sucking, high-pitched crying, fever, excessive yawning, and hyperreflexia.

Fetal Exposure Heroin

Heroin is a highly addictive, opioid narcotic that is a common drug of abuse. Heroin users are at increased risk of poor nutrition, iron deficiency anemia and preeclampsia-eclampsia, all negatively affecting the fetus. Infants with prenatal heroin exposure display symmetric intrauterine growth retardation (IUGR) and are often born prematurely. Sixty to 80 % of these infants will undergo neonatal abstinence syndrome (NAS). Heroin has a relatively short half-life and symptoms of NAR typically begin 48-72 hours after delivery. Several different body systems are affected by NAS and include:

CNS Dysfunction	GI Dysfunction	Miscellaneous Signs
High-pitched cry hyperactive. Reflexes increased muscle. Irritability. Tremors.	Poor feeding. Periods of frantic sucking or rooting. Vomiting. Loose or watery stools. Vomiting.	Frequent yawning. Sneezing multiple times. Sweating. Fever. Tachypnea.

Fetal Exposure Methadone

Methadone is commonly used to treat women who are addicted to heroin as it blocks withdrawal symptoms and drug craving, but methadone crosses the placental barrier and exposes the fetus to the drug. Many female heroin users are of reproductive age and methadone is often administered to pregnant women to decrease dangers associated with heroin, such as fluctuating levels of drug and exposure to hepatitis and HIV from sharing of needles. Exposure to methadone may result in miscarriage, stillbirth, intrauterine growth restriction, fetal distress, and low birth rate although symptoms are usually less severe than with heroin. However, if the mother takes methadone and other drugs, this can compound the adverse effects. Additionally, sudden withdrawal from methadone may cause preterm labor or death of the fetus, so methadone should be monitored carefully.

Fetal Exposure Cocaine

Cocaine/crack (freebase cocaine) is a nonopioid substance that readily crosses the placenta through simple diffusion. One of the most potent properties of cocaine is the ability of it to act as a vasoconstrictor. When a mother uses cocaine, the blood supply to the placenta is severely compromised when the vessels constrict, compromising blood flow and resulting in growth retardation and hypoxia. Cocaine also causes a programmed cell death (known as apoptosis) in the heart muscle cells of the fetus, resulting in cardiac dysfunction for the fetus. Maternal cocaine use increases the risk of premature birth and causes serious consequences for the neonate after birth. Maternal cocaine use can cause cerebral infarctions, nonduodenal intestinal atresia, anal atresia, NEC, defects of the limbs, and genitourinary defects. Cocaine stimulates the central nervous system by limiting the uptake of certain neurotransmitters norepinephrine, serotonin, and dopamine. Cocaine has a direct toxic effect on the nervous system, so the infant will exhibit extreme irritability and tremors followed by sluggish, lethargic behavior.

Fetal Exposure Common Prescription/OTC Drugs

Many **OTC and prescription drugs** have teratogenic effects on the developing fetus and can result in congenital abnormalities, growth retardation, intellectual disability, carcinogenesis, mutagenesis, and miscarriage. The degree of damage relates to multiple factors, such as the amount of drug reaching the fetus, the developmental period during which the drug is taken, and the duration. There are some recognizable syndromes:

- *Fetal warfarin (Coumadin®) syndrome* (exposure 7-12 weeks): Nasal hypoplasia, laryngomalacia, atrial septal defects, patent ductus arteriosis, eye, ear, and skull abnormalities, mental and growth retardation, brachydactyly, and scoliosis. Exposure during 2nd and 3rd trimester may result in eye abnormalities (cataracts, optic atrophy), microphthalmia (eyes stop developing resulting in abnormally small eyes), fetal/maternal hemorrhage, and microcephaly,
- *Fetal hydantoin (Dilantin®) syndrome* (exposure 1st trimester): Facial dysmorphism, microcephaly, underdeveloped nails (hands and feet), cleft left/palate, and developmental delays ranging from mild to severe.
- *Fetal valproate (Depakote®) syndrome* (exposure 1st trimester): Facial dysmorphism, spina bifida, CNS and cardiac abnormalities, and delay in development.

Continuation of **OTC and prescription drugs**, teratogenic effects (Part 2): Some drugs are classified as high risk (FDA classification D), but use is acceptable if the mother has a life-threatening illness or other drugs are not available, so neonates may exhibit adverse effects.

Drugs with high risk include and their adverse effects on the fetus/infant include:

- **ACE inhibitors** (2nd and 3rd trimesters): Skull and pulmonary hypoplasia, renal tubular dysplasia, and oligohydramnios.
- **Carbamazepine** (1st trimester): Craniofacial defects, neural tube defects, retardation of growth, and hypoplasia of fingernails.
- **Antineoplastic alkylating drugs** (1st to 3rd trimesters): Eye disorders, including microphthalmia and cataracts, cardiac defects, renal agenesis, and cardiac abnormalities.
- **Iodides** (3rd trimester): Thyroid disorders, including goiter, and fetal hypothyroidism.
- **Methimazole** (1st trimester): Aplasia cutis.
- **Lithium** (1st trimester): Ebstein's anomaly, various cardiac abnormalities.
- **Tetracycline** (2nd and 3rd trimesters): Yellow discoloration of teeth. Weakening of fetal bones and dysplasia of tooth enamel.

Continuation of **OTC and prescription drugs,** teratogenic effects (Part 3): Some drugs are classified as extremely high risk (FDA classification X), and these drugs should not be used with women who are pregnant or might become pregnant because fetal risk outweighs benefits to mother:

Agent	Greatest risk	Adverse effects on fetus/infant
Androgens	1st trimester (1-12 weeks)	Female fetus will become masculinized.
Retinoids (isotretinoin, acitretin, tretinoin, etretinate)	1st trimester	Multiple deformities of heart, ears, face, limbs, & liver, cognitive impairment, thymic hypoplasia, microcephalus, hydrocephalus, microtia, and miscarriage.
Thalidomide	Days 34-60	Multiple facial, intestinal, cardiac, limb abnormalities, including lack of limbs and limb reductions, and deafness.
Vitamin A >18,000 IU/day	Not established	Multiple craniofacial deformities, microtia, CAN and cardiac abnormalities, atresia of bowel, limb reductions, and defects of urinary tract.

Withdrawal Symptoms

Fetal exposure to drugs, such as opioids, methadone, cocaine, crack, and other recreational drugs, causes **withdrawal symptoms** in about 60% of infants. There are many variables, which include the type of drug, the extent of drug use, and the duration of maternal drug use. For example, children may have withdrawal symptoms within 48 hours for cocaine, heroin, and methamphetamine exposure, but there may be delays of up to 2 -3 weeks for methadone. Short hospital stays after birth make it imperative that children at risk are identified so they can receive supportive treatment, particularly since they often feed poorly and can quickly become dehydrated and undernourished. Polydrug use makes it difficult to describe a typical profile of *symptoms*, but they usually include:

- Tremors.
- Irritability.
- Hypertonicity.
- High-pitched crying.

- Diarrhea.
- Dry skin.
- Seizures (in severe cases).

Treatment is supportive, but children with opiate exposure may be given decreasing doses of opiates, such as morphine elixir, with close monitoring until the child is weaned off of the medication.

Dealing with Symptoms of Drug Exposure

Managing symptoms of **drug exposure**:

Symptoms	Intervention
High-pitched crying	Keep room quiet with low light. Swaddle the infant securely in a flexed position with the arms close to the body. Hold infant close to body. Rock swaddled infant slowly and rhythmically. Walk with swaddled infant held close. Offer pacifier, possibly with sugar solution if acceptable. Give a warm bath. Play soft music. Placing the infant in a dark room with no stimulation at all for a period of time may be effective if other methods fail.
Inability to sleep	Decrease environmental stimuli/ maintain quiet. Waterbed or sheepskin. Feed frequently in small amounts.
Nasal stuffiness sneezing	Aspirate nasopharynx as needed. Feed slowly and give time for rest between sucking. Monitor respirations.
Poor feeding and frantic sucking (fingers, fist)	Feed small frequent amounts with enteral feedings if necessary. Daily weight. Nonnutritive sucking with pacifier to relieve frantic sucking.
Regurgitation	Weigh frequently and monitor fluids and electrolytes. Observe for dehydration and provide IV fluids as needed. Place supine with head elevated after feedings.
Hypertonicity	Monitor temperature and decrease environmental temperature if infant's temperature >37.6°C. Change infant's position frequently to avoid pressure sores. Place on sheepskin or waterbed to prevent pressure.
Diarrhea	Change diaper frequently and cleanse skin with mild soap and water. Apply skin barrier as needed. Expose irritated skin to air.
Tremor, seizures	Decrease environmental stimuli and handling. Change position frequently. Observe for scratches, blistering, or abrasions. Place on sheepskin or waterbed to reduce friction and pressure. Maintain patent airway and observe for apnea. Monitor for hyperthermia.

Maternal Assessment: Antepartum Fetal Assessment

Fetal Lung Maturity

Tests for fetal lung maturity are important for monitoring fetuses if there is an indication for early termination of pregnancy. Pulmonary maturity is often an important factor is neonatal survival as immaturity can result in respiratory distress syndrome (RDS). Tests of amniotic fluid include:

- ***Lecithin/sphingomyelin (L/S) ratio:*** The ratio of the phospholipids lecithin and sphingomyelin (two components of surfactant) changes during pregnancy with L/S ratio at 0.5:1 early in pregnancy, 1:1 at 30-32 weeks, and 2:1 at 35 weeks. At 2:1, RDS is unlikely, although this finding is not always accurate for infants of diabetic mothers (IDM) as they may show adequate ratio but still develop RDS, so these neonates must be monitored carefully. This test is not accurate if the amniotic fluid contains blood or meconium.
- ***Phosphatidylglycerol (PG):*** This phospholipid first appears in surfactant at about week 35 in IDM with complications and week 36 in other pregnancies. Its presence is a sign of lung maturity.

Commonly, both tests are done to confirm lung maturity.

Ultrasound

Ultrasound uses high-frequency sound waves to produce images (sonograms) on a screen with fluid appearing black, soft tissue gray, and dense tissue (such as bone) black. A transducer turns the sounds waves into electrical signals and may be used transabdominally or transvaginally to evaluate the fetus:

- ***Transabdominal***: Done with full bladder to facilitate assessment of cervix, vagina, and bladder unless used to guide amniocentesis.
- ***Transvaginal***: Inserted into the vagina, this allows clearer images and better assessment of the cervix

Displays may show motion or be static. Ultrasounds may produce two-dimensional (B mode) or three-dimensional images and can be done in all 3 trimesters to determine position of the fetus, identify fetal anatomic structures, estimate fetal weight and/or growth, locate the placenta, determine presentation and viability of the fetus and/or multiple fetuses, guide amniocentesis, and determine the amniotic fluid index. Ultrasounds do not appear to pose a danger to the fetus or increase risk of miscarriage.

Amniocentesis

Amniocentesis is done at 15-20 weeks for genetic diagnoses and at 30-35 weeks to determine fetal lung maturity. Ultrasound locates the placenta and fetus and identifies an area with adequate amniotic fluid. The needle is inserted carefully to avoid major structures, the fetus, and arteries. A local anesthetic may be administered before insertion of a 22-gauge spinal needle into the uterine cavity. The first drops of fluid are discarded and a syringe attached. About 15-20 mL of amniotic fluid are withdrawn and placed in tubes, brown-tinted to shield the fluid from light that might break down bilirubin or other pigments. Ultrasound is again used to monitor removal of the needle, and the insertion point is checked for streaming (leakage of fluid). If the mother is Rh-negative, she is given Rh immune globulin immediately unless already sensitized. The fetal heart rate is monitored. Miscarriage occurs in about 1 in 200.   If performed at 11-14 weeks, there is increased risk to the fetus. Infection of the placenta (chorioamnionitis) is a rare complication.

Biophysical Profile

The **biophysical profile** comprises 5 measurements that are assessed to confirm the health of the fetus:

Measure: FHR

Explain: Measures fetal heart rate and acceleration with movement as measured by the nonstress test (NST). The NST is done during the daytime with the woman in semi-Fowler's position with support under right hip to displace the uterus to the left. Two monitors are applied to the abdomen—an ultrasound transducer to measure FHR and a tocodynamometer to detect fetal movement. The monitoring continues for 20-40 minutes (time extended if fetus appears to be in sleeping cycle). Occasional decelerations are normal, but repeated decelerations correlate with increased risk of Caesarean section. The woman reports sensations of fetal movement and this is compared to recording of movement. Correlation of 50-90% is normal.

Normal (Score 2): ≥ 2 FHR accelerations of 15 bmp above baseline for ≥15 seconds in a 20-40-minute period.

(Reactive)

Abnormal (0): 1-0 accelerations of FHR in 40 minutes.

(Nonreactive)

Measure	Normal (Score 2)	Abnormal (0)
Fetal respirations	≥ 1 episode of rhythmic breathing for ≥30 seconds in a 30-minute period.	≥30 seconds of rhythmic breathing in 30 minutes.
Fetal movement	≥ 3 separate movements in 30 minutes.	≥2 movements in 30 minutes.
Fetal tone	≥ 2 episodes of extension and flexion of arm/leg (or opening/closing of a hand)	No extension/flexion.

The 5 different measurements are completed and scores (2 for normal and 0 for abnormal) are compiled and interpreted according to risk for asphyxia. Maximum score is 10:

Score	Risk of Fetal Asphyxia	Discussion
10	Normal fetus with no risk.	No intervention indicated.
8	Little/rare risk to fetus.	No intervention indicated.
8 with abnormal amniotic fluid volume	Suspected chronic asphyxia.	Increased risk of perinatal mortality ≥ 1 week (89:1000), so birth should be induced.

6	Possible asphyxia.	Induce birth if amniotic fluid volume abnormal, if fluid level is normal at >36 weeks with cervix favorable, and if repeat test is ≥6. Observe and repeat tests according to protocol if repeat test is >6.
4	Possible asphyxia.	Induce birth if amniotic fluid volume abnormal, if fluid level is normal at >36 weeks with cervix favorable, and if repeat test is ≥6. Observe and repeat tests according to protocol if repeat test is >6.
2	Asphyxia virtually certain.	Marked increase in risk of perinatal mortality (125:1000), so birth should be induced.
0	Certain asphyxia.	Risk of perinatal mortality extremely high (600:1000), so birth should be induced.

Nonstress Test

The **nonstress test (NST)** measures fetal heart rate and acceleration with movement and is done during the daytime with the woman in semi-Fowler's position with support under the right hip to displace the uterus to the left. Two monitors are applied to the abdomen: an ultrasound transducer to measure FHR and a tocodynamometer to detect fetal movement. The monitoring continues for 20-40 minutes (time extended if fetus appears to be in sleeping cycle). Occasional decelerations are normal, but repeated decelerations correlate with increased risk of Caesarean section. The woman reports sensations of fetal movement, and this is compared to recording of movement. Correlation of 50-90% is normal.

Scoring:

- 2: Normal score with ≥ 2 FHR accelerations of 15 bmp above baseline for ≥15 seconds in a 20-40-minute period. (Reactive).
- 0: Abnormal score with 1-0 accelerations of FHR in 40 minutes. (Nonreactive).

Alpha-Fetoprotein

Alpha-fetoprotein (AFT) is a protein produced by the yolk sac for the first 6 weeks of gestation and then by the fetal liver. Cutoff levels have been established for each week of gestation, with peak levels at about week 15. The test is used primarily to detect neural tube defects (NTDs), which develop in the first trimester. AFT can be measured in amniotic fluid or maternal serum.

Triple screening includes *serum AFT level* done in the second trimester, and a positive result (which may be the result of errors in the duration of gestation) is followed by *ultrasound* and amniocentesis to check the *amniotic AFT level*. There is increased production of AFT with NTDs as well as abdominal wall defects and congenital nephrosis, so these levels can be used for assessment. (High quality ultrasound may also provide evidence of neural tube defects). The accuracy of tests varies depending upon the week of gestation. The most accurate results are acquired with testing during weeks 15-16.

Fetal Fibronectin Test

Fetal fibronectin (fFN) is a fetal extracellular glycoprotein that can be found in maternal cervical and vaginal secretions for the first 16 to 20 weeks of gestation, but then it is not found until near term. The fetal fibronectin test is one that is carried out to assess the risk of preterm birth. If an increase in fFN is noted, this may be an indication that preterm labor may start, although this is not always the case. False positives may occur with fetal or maternal infection, cervical manipulation before collection of specimen, sexual intercourse within 24 hours, lubricating gels, and vaginal bleeding. However, the absence of increased fFN almost always indicates that labor will not begin within the next 7 days. **Contraindications** include cervical dilation of ≥3 cm, suspected placental abruption or previa, vaginal bleeding, membrane rupture, or gestational age <22 weeks or >35 weeks. Special fFN kits are available for sample collection, which is taken with a speculum exam by rotating a swab across the vaginal fornix for 10 seconds and then inserting the swab into the collection tube.

Maternal Assessment: Intrapartum

Fetal Heart Rate Monitoring

Fetal heart rate (FHR) monitoring is usually done by electronic fetal monitoring (EFM) as it provides a continuous tracing. FHR can be assessed by *auscultation* or *ultrasound* with an abdominal transducer, but tracings can be poor with an active fetus, with maternal movement, and with hydramnios. *Internal monitoring* requires cervical dilation of ≥2cm so that an electrode can be applied to the fetal presenting part (head or buttocks). Internal scalp electrodes should not be used if the mother has a communicable disease, such as HIV, or with preterm infants. *Telemetry* with ultrasound or fetal ECG transducers and external uterine pressure transducers can also be used to monitor FHR. This type of battery-operated monitoring can be used while the mother ambulates, as it is less invasive. FHR patterns are evaluated based on a baseline rate (rate for 10 minutes between contractions), usually 110-160 bpm. Bradycardia is a rate <110 bmp; and tachycardia, >160 bpm.

Induction of Labor

Induction of labor stimulates uterine contractions to speed birth and may be done for many conditions, including diabetes mellitus, pre-eclampsia, post-term gestation, mild *abruptio placentae*, oligohydramnios, and poor biophysical profile. Induction is contraindicated with abnormal fetal heart rate patters, breech or uncertain presentation, multiple gestation, maternal heart disease or hypertension, and polyhydramnios. Common induction methods include:

- *Stripping/sweeping amniotic membrane:* A gloved finger is inserted through the cervical os and rotated (360°) two times to separate the amniotic membrane from the lower part of the uterus in order to release prostaglandins and stimulate contractions. Although not always effective, labor usually begins in 24-48 hours.
- *Oxytocin infusion:* Oxytocin (Pitocin®) is used to stimulate contractions of the uterus for induction of labor, but risks include over-stimulating the uterus, causing too frequent/intense contractions as well as uterine rupture, and water intoxication.
- *Complementary methods*: These methods include sexual intercourse, nipple stimulation, and herbal/homeopathic preparations. These methods have few negative effects.

Tocolysis

Tocolysis suppresses preterm labor and premature birth, sometimes allowing time to administer betamethasone to accelerate maturity of fetal lungs. Tocolytics (some off-label) include:

- **Nifedipine** a calcium channel blocker that reduces muscle contractility is most commonly used, as it is more effective and safer than many other drugs. It may increase fetal heart rate (FHR).
- **Terbutaline** is a β-adrenergic asthma drug that also relaxes the uterine muscle. It may increase FHR.
- **Magnesium sulfate** is similar in action to terbutaline, but it requires close monitoring for maternal adverse effects. It crosses the placenta, and the neonate may suffer respiratory and motor depression.
- **Indomethacin,** NSAID that inhibits prostaglandin production, can be used up to 32 weeks of gestation. It crosses the placenta and can cause reduction in amniotic fluid, leading to fetal distress, especially >32 weeks. Indomethacin can also cause premature closure of the ductus arteriosus.
- **Ritodrine** is a β-2 agonist that relaxes smooth muscles and can delay delivery for 24-48 hours but may increase fetal heart rate.

Effects of Opioids and Sedatives During Labor on Fetus/Neonate

Opioids and sedatives are usually given only in the early stages of labor, sometimes with PAC, because they readily cross the placental barrier and can cause central nervous system depression in the fetus. This depression can persist after delivery, especially in premature infants, affecting Apgar scores. Some drugs, such as morphine and benzodiazepines, are avoided because of excessive fetal depression. Drugs used include:

- **Meperidine** (1-25 mg IV or 25-50 IM to maximum 100 mg) is the most common. IV onset is 1-20 minutes and IM 1-3 hour, and its use is limited to >4 hours before delivery.
- **Fentanyl** (25-100 µg/hr IV) has shorter onset (3-10 minutes) with 1hour duration and causes less fetal depression, but may depress neonatal respirations.
- **Butorphanol** 1-2 mg or **nalbuphine** 10-20 mg IV or IM causes little respiratory effect and provides adequate relief of pain but may result in excessive sedation if given repeatedly.
- **Promethazine** (25-50 mg IM) and **hydroxyzine** may be used in combination with meperidine or alone to provide relief of anxiety and reduce dose of opioid.

Analgesia/Anesthesia (Epidural)

The most common form of regional anesthesia/analgesia for labor and delivery is the **lumbar epidural**. Dilute mixtures of local anesthetic and opioids are combined. The catheter is usually placed early so that it is in place when pain relief is needed. At one time, epidurals were delayed until labor was well established, but current trends are to administer earlier if the fetus is in no distress, contractions are 3-4 minutes and persisting at least 60 seconds, and the fetal head is engaged with 3-4 cm of cervical dilation. If dilute anesthetic agents are used, the mother may be able to ambulate while receiving the epidural. Fetal response relates to the drug used and the dosage, but can include abnormal fetal heart rate. If the mother becomes hypotensive from the drugs, this can reduce oxygen to the fetus and increase stress. After delivery, the neonate may exhibit increased incidence of hyperbilirubinemia, lethargy, decreased responsiveness, and depressed rooting and suckling reflex, leading to initial difficulty feeding.

Polyhydramnios

Polyhydramnios is increased amounts of amniotic fluid (>500 mL) present during fetal development and is associated with an elevated perinatal mortality rate. Approximately 25% of pregnant women with polyhydramnios experience preterm labor and delivery of a premature infant. Approximately 20% of infants born to mothers with polyhydramnios have an associated anomaly. Some conditions associated with polyhydramnios include:

- Obstructional lesions in the GI tract, such as duodenal atresia or tracheoesophageal fistula with esophageal atresia.
- Anencephaly.
- Central nervous system anomalies that impair the swallowing reflex.
- Cardiovascular rhythm anomalies associated with hydrops.
- Twin-twin transfusion syndrome in multiple pregnancies.
- Macrosomia.
- Fetal or neonatal hydrops.
- Chromosomal abnormalities such as trisomy 21, 18, or 13.
- Skeletal malformations such as congenital hip dislocation, clubfoot, or limb reduction.
- Increased risk for prolapsed umbilical cord and placental abruption.

Oligohydramnios

Oligohydramnios is decreased amounts of amniotic fluid (<500mL). Amniotic fluid cushions the fetus during development and is also necessary for normal development of the lungs. After 20 weeks of gestation, amniotic fluid is mainly produced by the fetus' excretion of urine. Fluids secreted by the respiratory tract and the oral/nasal cavity also contribute to the production of amniotic fluid. Oligohydramnios signals significant congenital pathology in the fetus and is associated with an elevated perinatal mortality rate. Some conditions associated with oligohydramnios include:

- Urinary tract anomalies:
  - o Obstructive uropathy.
  - o Renal agenesis.
  - o Polycystic kidneys.
- Pulmonary hypoplasia.
- Pressure deformities, such as clubbed feet.
- Compression of the umbilical cord, leading to fetal hypoxia.
- Meconium staining.
- Post term gestation.
- Leaking of amniotic fluid, prolonged or premature rupture of membranes, which are risk factors for neonatal infections.

Fetomaternal Hemorrhage and the Kleihauer-Betke Test

Fetomaternal hemorrhage (FMH) occurs in many pregnancies without any signs or symptoms. A small amount of fetal blood in the maternal circulation (1-2 ml) has no clinical significance. Massive FMH (blood loss greater than 30 ml) occurs in about 3 of every 1,000 pregnancies, and is a major cause of stillbirths. Neonates' blood volume ranges from 85-100 ml/kg, so 30 ml of blood loss represents 10-12% of the blood volume in a 3 kg neonate. Risk factors for FMH include maternal trauma, placental abruption, placental tumors, third trimester amniocentesis, fetal hydrops, and twinning. One test used to diagnose the presence of FMH is the Kleihauer-Betke (KB) test, in which a sample of the mother's blood is examined for the presence of fetal hemoglobin. The KB test estimates the amount of hemorrhage that has taken place.

Rupture of Membranes

Premature rupture of membranes (PROM): The amniotic sac breaks, ideally at term (40 weeks), prior to onset of labor. About 80% go into labor within 24 hours, and if labor doesn't commence in 12-24 hours, the patient must be frequently monitored until labor begins to ensure adequate amniotic fluid remains, or labor may be induced to prevent infection if the child is at term.

- *Spontaneous rupture (SROM)* usually occurs in the early stage of labor during an intense contraction, causing the fluid to gush out the vagina.
- *Preterm premature rupture of membranes (PPROM)* occurs in a woman <37 weeks of gestation and prior to the onset of labor. The patient is monitored as with premature rupture. It is one of the leading causes of premature birth.
- **Prolonged rupture of membranes**: ROM that persists for greater than 24 hours prior to the onset of labor. It is associated with increased risk of infection in the neonate.

Precipitous Labor/Birth

Precipitous labor birth and birth occurs when onset of labor to birth takes only ≥3 hours, often because of strong uterine contractions and low muscle resistance in maternal tissue that promotes rapid dilation of the cervix (or lacerations) and descent of the fetus. A primigravida may dilate 5 cm per hour; and a multigravida, 10 cm per hour. The neonate may have a low Apgar score and is at increased risk for aspiration of meconium and intracranial injury, such as subdural/dural tears. The strong uterine contractions may interfere with uterine blood flow and oxygenation of the fetus. Precipitous birth alone, by contrast, is usually an unexpected and sudden birth that takes place outside of the hospital or is unattended by a physician because there is no time to travel or get help. In these cases, the neonate is sometimes expelled into a toilet or onto the floor, causing injury.

Post-Term Pregnancy

Post-term pregnancy (>294 days or 42 weeks past 1st day of last menstrual period) occurs in 3-7% of pregnancies, and is often the result of errors in calculating due date, but true post-term pregnancies, while posing little risk to the mother, can increase risk to the fetus, and vaginal birth may be facilitated by forceps or vacuum extractor. Increased fetal risks include:

- *Large for gestational age* (LGA), >4500g (about 10 pounds), which may result in prolonged labor, birth trauma with fractures or neurological injury, or Caesarean section.
- *Aspiration of meconium* occurs more frequently because a large fetus is more likely to expel meconium.
- *Post-maturity syndrome* related to restriction of growth in the uterus, often because of restricted blood flow, putting the fetus at risk for respiratory and neurological disorders.

Multiple Gestations

In vitro fertilization and ovulation-inducing drugs have increased the incidence of high order **multiple gestations** over the past 30 years. The trend of delayed childbearing has led to an increase in twin/multiple gestations. Infants born from multiple gestations are more likely to be born prematurely and with low birth weights. The incidence of premature birth and low birth weight is proportional to the number of fetuses. There may be growth restriction/growth

- 33 -

discordance, oligohydramnios, and restriction of movement of one or more fetuses Approximately 50% of twins and 90% of triplets are born premature, compared to 10% of singletons. With this increase in prematurity and proportion of infants born with low birth weight, there are increased morbidities, such as cerebral palsy and intellectual disability. The risk for genetic disorders, such as neural tube defects, GI, and cardiac abnormalities, is twice that of single gestations.

Placenta Previa and Abruptio Placentae

Placenta previa: Implantation of the placenta is over or near the internal cervical os. Women with placenta previa have increased incidences of hemorrhage in the third trimester. In infants, placenta previa is associated with poor growth, anemia, and increased risk of congenital anomalies in their central nervous systems, heart, respiratory and gastrointestinal tracts. Placenta previa may also cause premature birth with associated neonatal complications of prematurity.

Abruptio placentae: The placenta prematurely detaches, partially or completely, from the uterine. Abruptio placentae is related to maternal hypertension and incidence increases with cocaine abuse. Partial detachment interferes with the functioning of the placenta, causing intrauterine growth retardation. Severe bleeding occurs with total detachment. Common fetal complications are preterm labor, hypoxia, and anemia. Fetal mortality is about 25% with partial detachment and 100% with complete. Irreversible brain damage may occur with fetal hypoxia, and neurological deficits occur in about 14% of survivors.

Prolapsed Umbilical Cord

A **prolapse of the umbilical cord** occurs when the umbilical cord precedes the fetus in the birth canal and becomes entrapped by the descending fetus. An ***occult cord prolapse*** occurs when the umbilical cord is beside or just ahead of the fetal head. About half occur in the second stage of labor and relate to premature delivery, multiple gestation, polyhydramnios, breech delivery, and an excessively long umbilical cord. Some cases are precipitated by obstetric interventions, such as amniotomy, external eversion, and application of scalp electrode for monitoring. As contractions occur and the head descends, this applies pressure to the umbilical cord, occluding blood flow and causing hypoxia and bradycardia. The decrease in blood flow through the umbilical vessels can cause impaired gas exchange, and if pressure on the cord is not relieved, the fetus can suffer severe neurological damage or death.

Cephalopelvic/Fetopelvic Disproportion

Cephalopelvic/fetopelvic disproportion is usually diagnosed when labor does not progress although in rare cases it may be diagnosed prior to labor. It may relate to pelvic diameters that are too small (most common with android and platypelloid pelvic types) or contractures of the pelvic inlet (<10 cm anteroposterior diameter or <12 cm transverse diameter), contracted midpelvis, or contracted outlet (<8 cm interischial tuberous diameter). Rarely is this disproportion caused by excessive fetal size as most fetuses are within normal size and weight limits. Usually labor is extended and premature rupture of the membranes occurs, increasing danger of cord prolapse. The fetal head is often markedly molded and continued pressure can cause neurological injury or even death of the fetus if the labor continues and the fetus cannot be delivered, but when labor fails to progress, the mother is usually given a Caesarean section (≥ 2 hours of labor onset) to prevent further injury to the fetus.

Fetal Malpresentation

Fetal malpresentation occurs when there is a variation in the normal cephalic (flexed neck) presentation during labor and delivery. There are 3 cephalic malpresentations:

- *Military*: The head is erect and neck not flexed, but his poses little problem because flexion often occurs as the head descends.
- *Brow:* The neck is extended so that the brow presents first. This presentation may relate to SGA, LGA, hydramnios, and uterine or fetal anomalies. Brow presentation, with the largest diameter (about 13.5cm), increases fetal mortality because of birth trauma, which can include compression of the neck and cerebrum and tracheal and laryngeal damage. Vaginal delivery with episiotomy or Caesarean is usually required.
- *Face*: The neck is severely extended so that the face presents first (about 9.5 cm diameter). This often prolongs labor and may result in increased edema of the fetus and trauma to the neck and internal structures. The neonate usually has bruising in the facial skin.

Additional **malpresentations** include:

- *Breech:* This occurs in 4% of births and is frequently related to early labor and delivery (25% at 25-26 weeks gestation). Frank breech (buttocks presentation with legs extended upward) is most common, but single or double footling breech or complete breech (buttocks presentation with legs flexed) can occur. Breech presentation is most common with placenta previa, hydramnios, fetal anomalies, and multiple gestation. Cord prolapse is more likely. Head trauma may occur because molding does not occur, and the head can become entrapped. Mortality and morbidity are reduced with Caesarean section, especially with low or high fetal weight, hyperextension of neck (>90°), fetal anomalies, and pelvic disproportion.
- *Shoulder:* This transverse lie poses extreme risk of uterine rupture. The fetus cannot be delivered, and Caesarean section is required.
- *Compound:* Two presenting parts, such as the head and a hand, increasing chances of laceration. With fetal distress or uterine dysfunction, Caesarean section is required.

Neonatal Assessment: Physical Assessment

Times and Types of Assessment

The neonate should undergo three different types of **physical assessment**:

- *Immediate*: The first examination is done in the delivery room to determine the need for resuscitation or other intervention. This includes APGAR assessment.
- *1-4 hours after birth:* The second examination includes gestational age assessment, which must be completed within 24 hours for accuracy, and brief physical assessment to determine if there are any problems that might place the infant at risk. This includes assessment of respiratory and cardiac status, cord color, skin color, and movement. The Modified Ballard scoring system is often used.
- *≥24 hours after birth (or prior to discharge):* The final examination should include a complete physical and behavioral assessment that includes all systems and evaluation of reflexes. All weights and measurements are taken and reviewed. This exam requires observation, palpation, and auscultation. In some cases, instead of a separate examination at 1-4 hours, only this complete physical examination is completed.

Head Assessment

The newborn has 8 skull bones and 14 facial bones. Their adjoining edges are bone sutures. Soft spots where the skull flexes along sutures to exit the vagina are **fontanels**. The newborn has 6 fontanels:

- Diamond-shaped anterior fontanel (AF): 2.1 cm.
- Triangular posterior fontanel (PF).
- Sphenoid fontanels (2).
- Mastoid fontanels (2).

The AF is the largest and most informative during clinical examination. Fontanels bulge when the newborn cries, vomits, lies down, or has hydrocephalus, intracranial tumor, hemorrhage, or meningitis. Fontanels should return to normal when the NNP holds the baby head up and the infant is calm. Depressed fontanels indicate the newborn is dehydrated. Conditions associated with an abnormally large AF include hypothyroidism, Down syndrome, achondroplasia, rickets, and increased intracranial pressure. Infants with Down syndrome may have an extra fontanel between the AF and posterior fontanel.

Craniotabes is an area of softened skull found in 30% of newborns. It is softer and more pliable than surrounding tissue and gives way when pressure is applied, as though one is pushing on a ping-pong ball. It is more common in premature infants, but can also be found in full term infants. Usually, craniotabes occurs in the posterior occipital or posterior parietal bones or along the suture lines. Craniotabes is considered to be a normal finding that requires no treatment because it usually resolves by one month of age. Craniotabes may persist longer when it is positioned along a suture line. No work-up is required, but the infant should be carefully examined for indications of disease-related causes of craniotabes, including other conditions that effect bone growth or hardness, such as rickets, syphilis, marasmus, or osteogenesis imperfecta.

Caput succedaneum and **cephalohematoma** are both examples of head molding resulting from head trauma during birthing. They can be observed during the newborn period and appear similar on physical examination because the neonate's head is swollen:

- *Caput succedaneum* is more common. It is a collection of fluid beneath the skin, but superficial to the periosteum. It often occurs when the head presses against the dilating cervix during the birth process. Vacuum assisted deliveries also contribute to caput succedaneum. The swelling crosses suture lines. Complications are rare. Swelling usually resolves over several days.
- *Cephalohematoma* occurs when blood vessels between the skull and the periosteum rupture, causing a subperiosteal collection of blood. The swelling appears several hours after birth. It does not cross suture lines. Complications such as anemia or hypovolemia may occur if the amount of bleeding is large. The blood will eventually be resorbed and may cause jaundice secondary to break down of red blood cells.

Eyes, Nose, and Neck Assessments

The appearance and movement of the **face** should be symmetric in the neonate and a number of different characteristics examined:

Eyes	Usually blue to blue/grey with white to bluish-white sclera. Small conjunctival hemorrhages and transient strabismus or squint may be evident. Pupils should be equal and reactive. Red retinal reflex should be present. Tears are usually absent during crying. Eye blink test causes lids to close.
Nose	Infants usually breathe through nose and should be able to breathe easily if mouth is closed. If not, the child should be examined for choanal atresia. Sense of smell is determined if the infant turns toward milk source or away from strong smells, such as alcohol.
Neck	The infant should be able to hold head up slightly while prone, but the head lags when lifted from the supine position because of weak muscles. Neck rigidity may indicate injury to sternocleidomastoid injury.

Mouth Assessment

The **mouth** should be carefully examined with a gloved finger pressing against the tongue to open the mouth:

Lips	Should be pink, normal-shaped, and symmetric. Thin upper lip with smooth philtrum and short palpebral fissures may indicate fetal alcohol syndrome.
Sucking	Sucking (symmetrical) should occur if lips are touched. Asymmetric movement of the mouth may indicate injury to facial nerve.
Gums	Examined for precocious teeth and Epstein's pearls (keratin-containing cysts).
Tongue	Examined for ridge of frenulum tissue on underside (tongue-tied) (although this is not clipped) and evidence of protrusion or hypertrophy, which can indicate various disorders, such as Down syndrome and hypothyroidism. Bluish swelling of the frenulum may indicate mucous/salivary gland retention cyst.
Mucous membranes	Examined for color and moisture as cyanosis may indicate respiratory distress and dryness, dehydration. Excessive salivation and drooling may indicate esophageal atresia. White patches on mucous membranes/tongue indicate infection with *Candida albicans*.

Ear Assessment

The ears should be carefully examined for a number of different characteristics:

Position	The insertion point of the top of the ear should be parallel to the inner and outer canthus of the eye. Low set ears may relate to a number of disorders, such as Trisomy 13 and Trisomy 18, intellectual disability, and various other disorders.
Shape/size	Ears should be proportionate to head size and symmetric.
Pliability	Ear should be soft and pliable. Cartilage is lacking in premature infants, and the pinna is soft. Cartilage should be firm by 38-40 weeks with 2/3 of pinna curving inward.

Hearing	Hearing may be initially assessed by observing response to sudden loud sound. Evoked otoacoustic emissions (EOAE) and auditory brainstem response (ABR) are used for universal hearing screening.
Tympanic membrane	Usually not examined with otoscope because of occlusion with vernix and blood after birth, but should appear gray-white and vascular.

Choanal Atresia

If the NNP is unable to pass a suctioning tube through the nares of the newborn, the infant may have **choanal atresia,** a rare condition that occurs in approximately 1 in 10,000 live births. It occurs in females twice as often as males. The choana are the two openings in the posterior nares that connect the nasal passages with the nasopharynx. Newborns are obligate nasal breathers. Successful nose breathing requires air to pass through the choana, so if these openings fail to form during fetal development, the infant must become a mouth breather. If atresia occurs only on one side (unilaterally), the infant may have no symptoms. The infant with bilateral choanal atresia has periods of respiratory distress and cyanosis that are alleviated by crying. Bilateral choanal atresia often becomes a medical emergency requiring intubation.

Chest and Respiratory Status

Chest/respiratory status should be evaluated by observation and auscultation. The chest should be symmetric, ribs flexible. The xiphoid process may protrude slightly, breasts are sometimes engorged, nipples may secrete small amounts of white fluid. Pulmonary function: includes anterior and posterior auscultation. Abdominal movement should synchronize with respirations. Periodic breathing is common; apneic periods should be <20 seconds. *Silverman-Anderson Index* evaluates respiratory status:

Characteristic	0	1	2
Chest/ abdomen	Rise together with inspiration	Abdomen rises, upper chest sinks	See-saw movement
Intercostals	No retraction	Minimal retraction	Pronounced retraction
Xiphoid process	No retraction	Minimal retraction	Pronounced retraction
Nasal flaring	None	Minimal	Pronounced
Grunt (expiratory)	None	Grunt heard with auscultation.	Audible grunt

Abdomen and Rectum Assessments

The **abdomen** should be soft, symmetric, and rounded. A distended abdomen with engorged vessels may indicate GI abnormalities. Bowel sounds (present about an hour after birth) should be auscultated prior to palpation. The liver is usually palpable 1-2 cm below right coastal margin, and the tip of the spleen may be palpable in preterm infants only in the left lateral upper quadrant (should not extend >1 cm below the costal margin). The umbilical cord should be white or blue-white with two umbilical arteries and one umbilical vein observed and no discharge or bleeding. Presence of only one umbilical artery is associated with GI/GU congenital anomalies. Green/yellow discoloration may indicate meconium staining. The abdomen should be examined carefully for hernias while the infant is at rest and crying.

The **rectal area** should be examined to determine if the anus is present and patent. Meconium is usually passed within 24 hours of birth. Soft swelling in the femoral area may indicate hernia or undescended testicle.

Back, Spine, and Extremities/Musculoskeletal System Assessments

The **back and spine** are examined with the infant in prone position. The spine should be straight without a sacral or lumbar curve (which develops after the child begins to sit). Obvious anomalies, such as spina bifida, and indications of a pilonidal dimple, skin lesions, or tufts of hair that may indicate abnormalities should be noted. C-shaped spine may indicate spina bifida occulta; and lumbar lordosis, myelomeningocele.

Extremities should be short, flexed, and able to move symmetrically through range of motion but without full extension.

The **musculoskeletal system** should be assessed for muscle tone. Maintenance of fetal position or limp tone may indicate hypoxia, CNS abnormalities, or hypoglycemia. Joint movement should be spontaneous with good muscle tone Spasticity or floppiness indicates cerebral palsy or other disorder. Jitteriness may indicate hypoglycemia or hypocalcemia. Arms/legs should be equal in length with feet and hands of normal size (5 digits each). Feet are flat. Hips should abduct to >60°. Cyanosis or clubbing of nails indicates cardiac anomalies; and yellow-green discoloration, meconium staining.

Male Genitalia Assessment

Male genitalia should be carefully examined to determine if they are clearly male or ambiguous:

Penis	The normal penis is usually about 2.5-3.5 cm long and 1 cm wide with the urinary meatus at the distal end in the glans. Displacement of the urethra is found with epispadias/hypospadias. Micropenis may indicate congenital anomaly. The urethral opening should not be inflamed. The foreskin should adhere to the glans and is tight (if uncircumcised). Small white cysts are sometimes evident on the prepuce.
Scrotum	Skin may be loose/hanging or tight/small with normal slightly darkened skin color and extensive rugae. A large scrotum should be examined by transillumination for hydrocele. If the skin is red and shiny, this may indicate orchitis. Discoloration (bruising) may be present with breech presentation.
Testes	Should be descended and 1.5-2cm in diameter, but may not be in scrotum and may be retractile (moving into the upper scrotum or inguinal canal on stimulation).

Hydrocele

A **hydrocele** is fluid in the scrotum or inguinal region. It co-occurs with an inguinal hernia in 10-20 infants per 1,000 live births. During fetal development, the testicles migrate from the abdominal cavity through the inguinal canal to the scrotum. A piece of peritoneum called the process vaginalis travels with the testicle into the scrotum. Normally, this extension of peritoneum closes and becomes a fibrous chord (tunica vaginalis), so there is no connection between the peritoneal cavity and the scrotum. If closure does not occur (patent process vaginalis), fluid accumulates in the scrotum. If the fluid collection comes and goes, then it is termed a communicating hydrocele. A non-communicating hydrocele is one where fluid is trapped in the scrotum after the process vaginalis closes. Physical examination reveals a bulge in the scrotum that may or may not be

reducible. No bowel sounds should be audible with auscultation, which indicates a hernia.
Transillumination of the scrotum reveals fluid retention.

Female Genitalia Assessment

Female genitalia should be assessed to determine·if there are indications of gender ambiguity as
enlarged clitoris and micropenis may be similar in appearance:

Mons	The labia majora should be symmetric and should cover the clitoris and labia minora in full-term and post-term infants although the labia minora and clitoris are exposed with preterm infants. The urinary meatus should be positioned below the clitoris. Bruising of the labia majora may be evident after vaginal birth.
Clitoris	The clitoris is enlarged in the neonate, and bruising and edema may occur with breech birth. Hypertrophy may indicate hermaphroditism.
Vagina	The vaginal opening should be evident (0.5cm). Hymenal tag may be observed in the vagina. White or pink-tinged vaginal discharge is common for 2-4 weeks after birth. An imperforate hymen may be indicated by suprapubic mass or mass between labia majora.

Newborn Skin Assessment

Skin colors vary with race, but all should be pink-tinged to some degree as skin pigmentation is
slight after birth. Skin characteristics include:

Birthmarks	Dark-skinned infants may have *Mongolian spots* on the buttocks and dorsal area. *Nevus flammeus* (port-wine stain) is a demarcated unraised red-purple lesion caused by capillaries below the epidermis. *Nevus vasculosus* (strawberry mark) is a capillary hemangioma and is a raised, demarcated dark red lesion.
Acro-cyanosis	Slight cyanosis of the hands and feet during the 2-6 hours after birth, especially if chilled. Color returns rapidly when skin blanched.
Mottling	Common for hours to weeks after birth and may relate to long periods of apnea/chilling.
Harlequin sign	Deep color on one side of body only for 1-20 minutes. Usually transient.
Erythema toxicum	Perifollicular lesions (1-3 mm) white or yellow with pustule appears suddenly over body (except palms and soles). Usually transient. Cause unknown.
Milia	Small raised white spots on face from exposed sebaceous glands. Transient.

Skin Appearance for the Pre-Term, Term, and Post-Term Neonate

Newborns' skin appearance depends on the development and thickening of their dermis,
epidermis, and vernix caseosa. When skin develops during week 15 of gestation, it is initially thin
and translucent. By week 20, vernix caseosa production begins. Vernix is a thick, waxy substance
secreted by the sebaceous glands and mixed with sloughed-off skin cells, often described as
"cheesy." The stratum corneum (protective top layer of the epidermis) develops from weeks 20-24.

The epidermis continues to develop and thicken, and is able to form a water barrier by week 32. Near term, the vernix washes away and the skin becomes more wrinkled without its protection:

Gestational Age	Skin Appearance
24-26 weeks	Translucent; red; many visible blood vessels; and scant vernix
35-40 weeks	Deep cracks; no visible blood vessels; and thick vernix
42-44 weeks	Dry, peeling skin; no vernix; and loss of subcutaneous fat

Café Au Lait Spots

Café au lait spots (CAL) are flat skin lesions with increased melanin content and regular or irregular borders. If the CAL spots are faint, one can use a Wood lamp to make them easier to see. Less than 3 café au lait spots have no clinical significance. However, 6 or more café au lait spots with a diameter larger than 5 mm occur in 95% of patients with neurofibromatosis type 1 (NF1), a disorder of chromosome 17. Lisch nodules on the child's iris and Crowe's sign (freckles on the axilla and inguinal area) corroborate the diagnosis of NF1. The pediatrician must be alerted that this child should receive future monitoring for the symptoms that occur with NF1, such as bowed legs, rib lesions, scoliosis, neurofibromas, glaucoma, and corneal opacification. Café au lait spots are also associated with Tuberous sclerosis, McCune-Albright syndrome, ataxia telangiectasia, Gaucher disease, basal cell nevus syndrome, and Fanconi anemia. Eighteen percent of infants affected with CAL are blacks, 3% are Hispanics, and 0.3% are whites.

Jaundice

Jaundice is yellowing of the skin and sclera (eye whites), indicating elevated bilirubin levels (hyperbilirubinemia). Elevated bilirubin levels occur normally during the newborn period because of the rapid breakdown of fetal hemoglobin after birth and the immaturity of enzymatic pathways in the newborn's liver (the organ responsible for metabolizing bilirubin). Physiological jaundice describes this normal process, which usually becomes evident on the second or third day of life by yellowing of the face. As bilirubin levels increase, the trunk and extremities become involved, and the skin yellows. The baby's eyes are covered and the baby placed in under blue lights (phototherapy). For most infants, jaundice is transient and resolves within a few days. Persistent or pronounced jaundice may indicate that further diagnostic testing or intervention is needed.

Appearance, Weight, Measurements, and Vital Signs

The neonate's general **appearance, measurements, and VS** should be evaluated:

- **Head:** Disproportionately large for body.
- **Body:** Long.
- **Extremities:** Short and in flexed position. (Feet usually dorsiflexed after breech birth.) **Hands:** Clenched.
- **Neck:** Short and chin resting on chest.
- **Abdomen:** Prominent **Hips:** Narrow **Chest:** Rounded.
- **Weight:** 2500-4000 g (average about 3400). Physiologic weight loss is 5-10% for full term and 155 for preterm.
- **Length:** 45-55 cm (average 50 cm).
- **Head circumference:** 32-38 cm (usually 2 cm greater than chest circumference).
- Chest circumference: 30-36 cm.

- **Temperature:** Temperature drops rapidly (skin temperature falls 0.3°C/minute) after birth with exposure to ambient room temperature but stabilizes within 8-12 hours. Temperature is usually measured by axillary method (for 3 minutes) and ranges from 36.3°C to 37.0°C.
- **Blood pressure:** 56-77/33-50 mm Hg.
- **Pulse:** 120-120 bpm awake; 100 bpm asleep; 180 bmp crying.
- **Respiration:** 30-60 per minute.

Infant Blood Pressure

Normal **blood pressure** values for *term infant:*

- Systolic-56-77 mm Hg.
- Diastolic 33-50 mm Hg.
- MAP 42-60 mm Hg.
- Hypertension: Systolic >90 and diastolic >60.

Normal values for ***preterm infant:*** In a preterm infant, systolic and diastolic values will vary depending on the gestational age and size of the infant. A preterm infant should have a mean arterial pressure that is a number matching the gestational age in weeks of that infant. For example, an infant born at 28 weeks gestation should have a MAP of 28.

- Hypertension: Systolic > 80 and diastolic >50.

Proper fit of the blood pressure cuff is imperative to obtain an accurate reading. One must measure the width of the infant's arm in the area that the cuff will be applied. Once this measurement is obtained, the cuff should be approximately 25% wider than this measurement. A cuff too small results in BP reading too high and too large results in BP reading too low.

Assessing Heart Sounds

S1 is the heart sound heard as the mitral and tricuspid valves close at the beginning of the contraction of the ventricle (systole). S1 is easiest to hear if the stethoscope is placed at the fourth intercostal space while the infant is supine and calm. If the S1 heard is louder than normal, that means cardiac output and blood flow are higher than normal. The conditions that can cause this are:

- Patent ductus arteriosis.
- Ventricular septal defect.
- Tetralogy of Fallot.

If the S1 heard is softer or quieter than normal, this is an indication of lowered cardiac output. The conditions that could cause this are:

- Congestive heart failure.
- Myocarditis.

S2 is the sound heard when the pulmonic valve and the aortic valve close at the end of the contraction of the ventricles (systole). S2 is easiest to hear at the upper left border of the sternum. S2 is normally split as the aortic valve closes slightly ahead of the pulmonic valve. In the presence of a cardiac defect, the S2 split becomes more far apart or widened (the difference in time between the closing of the aortic and pulmonic valve becomes greater). Conditions that cause a widened S2 split include:

- Atrial Septal Defect.
- Tetralogy of Fallot.
- Pulmonary Stenosis.
- Ebstein Anomaly.

Conditions that cause no split in the S2 (the two valves close at the same time or one is not closing) include:

- Pulmonary or aortic atresia.
- Aortic or Pulmonary stenosis.
- Persistent Pulmonary Hypertension.

Peripheral Pulses

Peripheral pulses are graded according to strength, usually palpated at the brachial or femoral arteries. However, peripheral pulses may be difficult to palpate in a neonate and should not be relied upon for cardiac assessment. Pulses should always be verified by auscultation:

0   = absent
1+ = weak
2+ = weak to average
3+ = strong
4+ = bounding

Weak pulses are noted in conditions that cause a decrease in cardiac output, some of these conditions include:

- Any defect resulting in obstructed blood flow leaving the left ventricle.
- Failure of the heart muscle itself.
- Shock.

Bounding pulses (4+) are noted when there is too much blood coming from the aorta, some of the conditions that would cause this are:

- Patent ductus arteriosus.
- Aortic insufficiency.
- Shunts.

Neonatal Assessment: Gestational Age

Modified Ballard Score

The **Modified Ballard Score** is used to estimate maturity and gestational age in newborn infants. It is most reliable when performed within the first 12 hours of life. The Ballard Score was modified to include evaluation of extremely premature infants with gestational ages as low as 20 weeks (score - 10) and as high as 50 weeks (score 44). It scores 6 measurements of neuromuscular maturity and 6

- 43 -

signs of physical maturity on a scale of -1 to 4 or 5 (depending upon the category). The total score indicates the estimated gestational age for that infant:

Neuromuscular Measurements	Physical Signs of Maturity
Supine posture	Skin characteristics
Square window (wrist)	Presence or absence of lanugo.
Arm recoil	Appearance of plantar feet surfaces.
Popliteal angle	Presence or absence of breast buds.
Scarf sign	Eye and ear characteristics.
Heel to ear	Genitalia (male and female) characteristics.

Neuromuscular measurements for **Modified Ballard Score:**

- Observation of the ***infant's posture*** while lying supine indicates the total amount of muscle tone the infant possesses. Increased amounts of flexion of the elbows and knees correlates with increased gestational age.
- ***Square window test*** measures the resistance to stretching of extensor muscles in the infant's forearm. Increased ability for the tester to flex the infant's wrist correlates with greater gestational age.
- ***Arm recoil test*** measures the tone of the biceps muscles. Increased amount of arm recoil (flexion by the infant after the infant's arms are extended) correlates with greater gestational age.
- ***Popliteal angle*** measurement assesses the flexor tone of the knee joint. Increased resistance to flexion at the knee is associated with greater gestational age.
- ***Scarf sign test*** measures the tone of shoulder flexor muscles. Increased resistance to movement of the infant's arm across the chest is associated with greater gestational age.
- ***Heel to ear test*** measures the tone of pelvic girdle muscles. Increased resistance to movement of the infant's foot to its ear is associated with greater gestational age.

Physical signs of maturity in the **Modified Ballard Score:**

- ***Skin***: Immature infants have thin, transparent skin. The vernix caseosa begins development at the beginning of the third trimester. Dried, cracked skin occurs as this protective coating disappears after the 40th week.
- ***Lanugo***: Fine, usually unpigmented hairs begin to appear at 24-25 weeks of gestation and thin as the neonate matures.
- ***Plantar surface of feet***: Very immature infants have no creases on the soles of their feet. Creases develop first on the anterior portion and more mature infants will have creases over the entire sole.
- ***Breast buds***: Fatty tissue underneath the areola that increases in size as the fetus matures.
- ***Ears***: Increased cartilage content produces a more rigid pinna; ear recoil increases as the infant matures.
- ***Male Genitalia***: The testes descend from the abdomen into the scrotum at 30 weeks of gestation and the scrotum develops rugae as the fetus matures.
- ***Female Genitalia***: Initially, the female fetus has a large clitoris and small labia majora. As the fetus matures, the labia majora enlarge, while the clitoris shrinks.

Infant Born at 24-25 Weeks

The Modified Ballard Score is used to accurately determine the gestational age of extremely premature infants. Infants born at **24-25 weeks gestational age** will have:

Characteristic	Expected findings
Skin	Very thin with visible veins. Absent or minimal vernix caseosa as it is just beginning to be secreted at 2weeks.
Lanugo	Sparse.
Feet	Smooth plantar surfaces or faint marks on the anterior surfaces.
Areolae	Newly developing, breast bud not yet present.
Eyes	Open.
Ears	No or very limited recoil.
Posture	Immature, indicated by limited flexion of the limbs while infant in supine position.
Square window sign	Shows decreased flexion at the wrist of approximately 60-90°.
Range of motion	Increased ROM (lone tone) when performing the popliteal angle, scarf sign, and heel to ear examinations.
Arm recoil	Limited or no recoil.

Preterm Infant

A **preterm** infant is one born prior to 37 weeks gestational age. In the United States, preterm birth is the most important factor influencing infant mortality; preterm infants account for 75-80% of all neonatal morbidity and mortality. Health problems associated with premature birth include:

- Respiratory distress syndrome because of inadequate surfactant production (hyaline membrane disease).
- Hypothermia because of inadequate subcutaneous fat, small amounts of brown fat, and large skin surface area to mass ratio.
- Hypoglycemia secondary to poor nutritional intake, poor nutritional stores, and increased glucose consumption associated with sepsis.
- Skin trauma or infection secondary to fragile, immature skin.
- Periods of apnea because of an immature respiratory center in the brain.
- Intraventricular hemorrhage.

The original cause of the preterm birth (such as maternal infection) may also play an integral role in the likely health problem associated with prematurity.

Neuromuscular Characteristics of a Full-Term Infant

Neuromuscular characteristics of a **full term (40-week) infant**:

Test	Result
Supine Resting Posture	Hips, knees, and arms all flexed past 90°, indicating mature muscular tone.
Square Window	The wrist flexes to 0°, reflecting very little resistance to the extensor muscles of the wrist.
Arm Recoil	Arms recoil past 90°. Contact between the infant's fist and face demonstrates mature tone in the biceps muscles.

Test	Result
Popliteal angle	<90° knee flexion.
Scarf Sign	The arms cannot be drawn past the ipsilateral axillary line because of the mature tone of the posterior shoulder girdle flexor muscles.
Heel to Ear	Resistance is felt in the knee and hip when the heel is at the femoral crease because of the tone of the posterior pelvic girdle flexor muscles.

Postterm Infant

Postterm infants are those born >42 weeks of gestation. Many are normal in size and appearance but some continue to grow *in utero* and weigh >4000 g and may exhibit postmaturity syndrome (about 5%), putting the infant at increased risk. Characteristics include:

- Alert *appearance* (may indicated intrauterine hypoxia).
- *Skin*: loose, dry, cracking, parchment-like, lacking lanugo or vernix. May have meconium staining—yellow to green (indicating recent).
- *Fingernails*: long (sometimes with meconium staining).
- *Scalp hair*: long/thick.
- *Body*: long, thin (fat layers absent).
- *Hypoglycemia* from nutritional deprivation.
- *Hypothermia* because of decreased brown fat and liver glycogen
- *Meconium aspiration* (risk increases with oligohydramnios), increasing risk of impaired gas exchange.
- *Polycythemia* as response to hypoxia, increasing risk of impaired tissue perfusion.
- *Seizures* resulting from hypoxia.
- *Cold stress* (lack of fat stores).
- Congenital anomalies.

Acronyms for Gestational Age

These terms do not take into account the estimated gestational age of the infant:

- **ELBW** (**E**xtremely **l**ow **b**irth **w**eight): Any infant with a birth weight of less than 1,000 g (2.2 lbs).
- **VLBW** (**V**ery **l**ow **b**irth **w**eight): Any infant with a birth weight of less than 1,500 grams (3.3 lbs.

The following terms take into account the estimated gestational age of the infant in comparison to the birth weight:

- **SGA** (**S**mall for **g**estational **a**ge): The birth weight of the infant is less than the 10th percentile for his or her gestational age.
- **AGA** (**A**ppropriate for **g**estational **a**ge): The birth weight of the infant is between the 10th and 90th percentile for his or her gestational age.
- **LGA** (**L**arge for **g**estational **a**ge): The birth weight of the infant is greater than the 90th percentile for his or her gestational age.

Large for Gestational Age (LGA)

Large for gestational age (LGA) infants are those whose weight places them above the 90th percentile for their gestational age. The main pathologic cause for LGA is maternal diabetes (either gestational diabetes or diabetes mellitus). Infants exposed to elevated levels of glucose produce elevated amounts of insulin, which has an anabolic effect on the developing fetus, causing macrosomia (large body). Poor control of diabetes during pregnancy generally results in a larger infant with these common health problems:

- Delivery complications (shoulder dystocia, clavicle fracture, prolonged vaginal exit requiring use of forceps or Caesarian section, and perinatal asphyxia).
- Abnormal blood test results (hypoglycemia developing within 1-2 hours of birth, hyperbilirubinemia, hypocalcemia, hypomagnesemia, hyperviscosity [thickened blood] secondary to polycythemia [elevated platelets]).
- Jaundice.
- Feeding intolerance.
- Lethargy.
- Respiratory distress.
- Birth defects.

Small for Gestational Age (SGA)

Small for gestational age (SGA) infants are those whose weight places them below the 10th percentile for their gestational age. SGA is also called dysmaturity and intrauterine growth restriction. SGA babies commonly aspirate meconium, and have a low APGAR score, asphyxia, hypoglycemia, and polycythemia. Common causes of SGA include:

- Multiple gestation (twins, triplets, quadruplets).
- Constitutional SGA because both parents are small.
- Many genetic defects, such as trisomy 18 (Edwards syndrome), Down syndrome, and Turner syndrome.
- Placental malfunction or misplacement (inadequate fetal nutrition from reduced blood flow, sepsis, placenta previa, or abruptio placentae).
- Maternal disease (pre-eclampsia; high blood pressure; malnutrition; advanced diabetes mellitus; chronic kidney, heart, or respiratory disease; and anemia).
- Infections such as cytomegalovirus, toxoplasmosis, and rubella.
- Maternal tobacco, illegal drug, or alcohol use during pregnancy.
- Birth defects.

Intrauterine Growth Restriction (IUGR)

When an infant does not fulfill his or her growth potential for any reason, the diagnosis is **intrauterine growth restriction** (IUGR). Prenatal ultrasound is used to diagnose IUGR, which is associated with oligohydramnios (decreased amniotic fluid) and pre-eclampsia (pregnancy-induced hypertension and proteinuria). IUGR is classified as symmetric or asymmetric, based on the size of the newborn's head:

Symmetric IUGR	Asymmetric IUGR
Both head and body are small (growth-restricted). Occurs early in pregnancy. Common causes are chromosomal abnormalities and infections.	Large head in proportion to the body; the head is spared. The head is normal in size for gestational age, while the body is growth-restricted. Occurs late in pregnancy. Common causes include placental insufficiency and preeclampsia.

Neonatal Assessment: Behavioral and Neurosensory

Brazelton Neonatal Behavioral Assessment Scale.

The **Brazelton Neonatal Behavioral Assessment Scale** is a multi-dimensional scale that is used to assess a neonate's state, temperament, and behavioral patterns. It includes assessment of 18 reflexes, 28 behaviors, and 6 other characteristics. It is usually completed on day 3 with an attempt to elicit the most positive response, usually when the infant is comforted and in a quiet dim room. Scoring correlates to the child's awake or sleep state. Infants are scored according to response in many areas, including:

- *Habituation*: Ability to diminish response to repeat stimuli.
- *Visual and auditory orientation:* Ability to respond to stimuli, fixate, and follow a visual object.
- *Motor activity:* Assessment of body tone in various activities.
- Variations: Changes in color, state, activity, alertness, and excitement during the exam.
- *Self-quieting activities:* Frequency and speed of self-calming activities, such as sucking on hand, putting hand to mouth, focusing on object or sound.
- *Social behaviors:* Ability to cuddle, engage, and enjoy physical contact.

Sleep States

Infants spend a high percentage of their time in **sleep states**. Sleep periods are divided into active sleep or quiet sleep by observing the infant's behavior:

- *Quiet sleep* is restorative and fosters anabolic growth. Quiet sleep is associated with increased cell mitosis and replication, lowered oxygen consumption, and the release of growth hormone. During quiet sleep, the infant appears relaxed, moves minimally, and breathes smoothly and regularly. The eyelids are still. The infant only responds to intense stimuli during quiet sleep.
- *Active sleep* is associated with processing and storing of information. Rapid eye movement (REM sleep) occurs during active sleep, but it is unknown if newborn infants are able to dream. During active sleep, the infant moves occasionally and breathes irregularly. Eye movements can be seen beneath the eyelids. Infants spend most of their sleep time in active sleep, and it usually precedes wakening.

Awake States

Infants have different levels of consciousness in the 4 **awake states**. Infants respond differently to outside stimuli and interaction from caregivers, depending on which state they are in:

- *Drowsy:* This is characterized by variable activity, mild startles, and smooth movement. There is some facial movement. Eyes open and close, breathing is irregular, and response to stimuli may be delayed.
- *Quiet alert:* The infant rarely moves, breathing is regular, and the infant focuses intently on individuals or objects that are within focal range, widening eyes. Face appears bright and alert, breathing is regular, and the infant focuses on stimuli.
- *Active alert:* The infant moves frequently and has much facial movement although face not as bright and alert, eyes may have a dull glaze, breathing is irregular, and there are variable responses to outside stimuli.
- *Crying:* Characterized by grimacing, eyes shut, irregular breathing, increased movement with color changes and marked response to both internal and external stimuli.

Autonomic Response

The neonate has an **autonomic response** to stress, especially auditory stimuli, so neonatal units must make efforts to reduce noise levels to <45 dB. It is especially important that physical assessment take place when the baby is not stressed, so the environment should be quiet with dim lights. Typical autonomic physiological responses to noise or other stress includes:

- Lability of states.
- Increased avoidance behaviors (startle, crying).
- Increased heart rate (often initially) and bradycardia.
- Increased respiratory rate or apnea.
- Increased hypoxemia.
- Peripheral and arterial vasoconstriction with increased BP and ICP (increasing risk of intraventricular hemorrhage).

These responses cause alterations of sleep cycles with increased periods of wakefulness and agitation, interfere with habituation, and decrease approach behaviors. Additionally, infants exposed to auditory stress may develop sensorineural hearing loss and abnormal auditory processing.

Neurosensory Capabilities

The **neurosensory capabilities** of the neonate are more acute than many people are aware:

- *Hearing*: The neonate's crying after birth clears middle ear mucous and the eustachian tubes, and hearing becomes acute with hearing thresholds similar to adults and children. Because hearing deficit is one of the most common congenital abnormalities, all infants should be assessed for hearing.
- *Vision*: The neonate's vision is about 10-30 times less acute than that of an adult, but the infant has peripheral vision and can fixate at 8-14 inches and can accommodate to large objects. The neonate is able to perceive shapes, colors, and faces.
- *Tactile sense:* The neonate has a good sense of touch and reacts emotionally to tactile stimulation.

- 49 -

- **Smell**: The neonate has a strong sense of smell after nasal passages clear and will react to the smell of milk or turn away from strong smells.
- **Pain**: Neonates experience pain, and pain prevention/management should be part of neonatal care.

Assessment of Muscular Tone

Determining the quality of **muscle tone** in a neonate is an important part of neuromuscular assessment. The child is placed supine with the head in neutral position and the NNP moves body parts (arms, legs, head) to determine if the muscle tone is flaccid, jittery, or hypertonic. Neonates are slightly hypertonic so that some resistance should be felt to movement, such as when moving a leg or straightening an arm. Tone should be symmetric. The extremities are usually flexed and legs abducted to abdomen. This assessment allows the NNP to differentiate common fine tremors or jitteriness found in neonates from seizure activity or nervous system disorders that cause muscular twitching. Normal fine tremors are usually halted by holding or flexing the extremity while seizure activity or twitching does not resolve by holding.

Assessment of Reflexes

Common neonatal **reflexes** include:

Reflex	Eliciting reflex	Normal Response	Discussion
Palmar Grasping	Stroke the infant's palm.	The infant responds by grasping your finger.	Grasp reflex is stronger in premature infants and fades away at 2-3 months of age. Absence indicates CNS deficit or muscle injury.
Rooting	Stroke the side of the infant's cheek.	The infant turns his/her head in the same direction as your touch, and opens his/her mouth to feed.	Rooting reflex helps the infant find and latch onto his/her mother's breast.
Sucking	Touch the infant's mouth.	The infant sucks.	Premature infants may have an absent or weak suck reflex, as it usually develops around week 32 of gestation. Weak or absent reflex indicates CNS deficit or depression.
Moro (Startle)	Make a loud sound or give the infant a gentle jolt.	The infant extends his/her arms, legs, and neck, and then pulls back his/her arms and legs. He/she may also cry.	Moro reflex disappears at 5-6 months of age. Asymmetric response indicates peripheral nerve injury, fractures (long bones, clavicle, or skull).
Blinking	Flash light at eyes.	Eyelids close.	Absence or delay may indicate cerebral palsy, hydrocephalus, and developmental delay.
Tonic neck (fencing)	With infant supine, turn head to one side.	Extremities flex on opposite side and extend on same side.	May be incomplete immediately after birth and should diminish by 4 months. Persistence >4 months may indicate neurological abnormalities.

Reflex	Eliciting reflex	Normal Response	Discussion
Babinski (plantar)	Stroke the lateral aspect of the sole from heel to ball of foot.	Hyperextension of all toes.	Persists until ≥2 years after which the toes flex.
Trunk incurvation (Galant)	With infant prone, stroke down one side of the spine (1 inch from spine)	Pelvis turns to stimulated side.	Absence indicates CNS depression or lesion of spinal cord. Should disappear by 4 months.

Assessment of the Sucking Reflex

Touching the roof of the neonate's mouth triggers **sucking**. The sucking reflex begins to appear at 32 weeks of gestation, but is not fully developed until 36 weeks. Premature neonates often have an immature or weak suck, and need additional patience and support to feed. Preterm neonates have difficulty coordinating sucking, swallowing and breathing simultaneously. Preterm neonates have immature neurological systems and less ability to handle external environmental stressors. Stressors include medically necessary and unavoidable frequent examinations, respiratory support from oxygen or a ventilator, administration of medications, light, noises of a busy NICU, or even oral feeds. As a neonate matures, the infants develop skills to self-soothe h when stressed. Some of these skills include nonnutritive sucking:

- Sucking of hands or fingers.
- Sucking on a pacifier.
- Sucking during sleep.

Neonatal Assessment: Clinical Laboratory Tests

Microbiological Testing

Neonates with exposure to microbiological agents before, during, or after birth may require **microbiological testing**:

- Blood cultures are done to isolate causative agents in order to begin appropriate antibiotic treatment.
- In some cases, microbiological testing of expressed breast milk may be indicated.
- Microscopic examination of urine and urine culture may be done to identify urinary pathogens.
- Stool cultures may be done to identify GI pathogens.
- Tracheal secretions may be cultured to identify pathogens causing pneumonia, especially in infants who are ventilated. The findings should be reviewed along with chest radiographs to ensure that positive findings don't just represent tracheal colonization alone.
- Gram stain and scraping of conjunctiva may be done to identify gonococcal conjunctivitis.
- Skin culture may be indicated for the infant with a skin infection.

Clinical Laboratory Tests for Electrolytes

Fluid and electrolyte balance must be maintained in the neonate. Fluid needs are usually estimated at 100 ml/kg but this may vary with changes in metabolic rate and output.

Calcium Normal Values:

- Cord: 8.2-11.2 mg/dL
- 0-10 days: 17.6-10.4 mg/dL
- 11 days-2 years: 9.0-11.0 mg/Dl

Discussion: Hypocalcemia: < 7 mg/dL is common with infants that are critically ill, IDM, suffered from asphyxia, or are preterm with very low birth weight.

Sodium Normal Values:

- Neonate: 133-146 mEq/L

Discussion: Hypernatremia: >150 mEq/L usually relates to dehydration, use of Na containing solutions, congenital or acquired reduction in ADH, cerebral palsy, and intracranial hemorrhage. Hyponatremia: <130 mEq/L usually relates to overhydration, renal excretion from diuresis, or SIADH.

Potassium Normal Values:

- Neonate: 2.7-5.9 mEq/L

Discussion:

Hyperkalemia: >7 mEq/L may relate to renal failure, acidosis, or adrenal insufficiency. Hypokalemia: <3.5 mEq/L usually relates to excessive GI or renal fluid losses.

Clinical Laboratory Urine Tests

Urine testing includes:

- *pH* should range from 4.5 to 9.0. An alkaline (high) pH can be caused by urinary tract infections, diarrhea, or kidney infection. An acidic (low) pH may reflect lung disease, hyperglycemia, or diarrhea with dehydration.
- *Specific gravity* ranges from 1.001 to 1.040 (usually about 1.015).

About 2% of full-term infants have asymptomatic bacteriuria, but this increases to about 10% for preterm infants. However, the urinalysis alone is not an effective test to determine if an infant has a urinary tract infection because the neonate's urine usually contains leukocytes (≥25/mm3 in males and ≥50/mm3 in females), and urine cultures of infants <3 days often show poor results, even in the presence of infection, so blood cultures (and in some cases cultures of CSF) should be done if infection is suspected as neonates are more likely to develop kidney infections and sepsis from cystitis than older infants. The most common infective agent is *Escherichia coli* although *Candida* and *Staphylococcus* are common with prolonged hospitalization.

Clinical Laboratory Tests for Arterial Blood Gases (ABGs)

Arterial blood gases (ABGs) are monitored to assess effectiveness of oxygenation, ventilation, and acid-base status, and to determine oxygen flow rates. Partial pressure of a gas is that exerted by each gas in a mixture of gases, proportional to its concentration, based on total atmospheric pressure of 760 mm Hg at sea level. Normal values for children include:

- Acidity/alkalinity (pH): 7.26-7.44.
- Partial pressure of carbon dioxide (PaCO$_2$): 35-45 mm Hg.
- Partial pressure of oxygen (PaO$_2$): >80 mg Hg.
- Bicarbonate concentration (HCO$_3$): 22-28 mEq/L.
- Oxygen saturation (SaO$_2$): >92-95%.

The relationship between these elements, particularly the PaCO$_2$ and the PaO$_2$ indicates respiratory status. For example, PaCO$_2$ >55 and the PaO$_2$ <60 in an infant previously in good health indicates respiratory failure. There are many issues to consider. Ventilator management may require a higher PaCO$_2$ to prevent barotrauma and a lower PaO$_2$ to reduce oxygen toxicity. Premature infants may need lower PaO$_2$ to prevent retinopathy of prematurity.

Additional Clinical Laboratory

Red Blood Cells

Red blood cells (RBCs or erythrocytes) are biconcave disks that contain hemoglobin (95% of mass), which carries oxygen throughout the body. The heme portion of the cell contains iron, which binds to the oxygen. RBCs live about 120 days in adults but this is reduced 20-25% in neonates and 50% in preterm infants. The RBCs are destroyed and their hemoglobin is recycled or excreted.

Normal values of red blood cell count vary by age:

- Neonate:4.1-6.1 million per mm^3.
- 2-6 mos:3.8-5.6 million per mm^3.

The most common disorders of RBCs are those that interfere with production, leading to various types of anemia:

- Blood loss.
- Hemolysis.
- Bone marrow failure.

The morphology of RBCs may vary depending upon the type of anemia:

- Size: Normocytes, microcytes, macrocytes.
- Shape: Spherocytes (round), poikilocytes (irregular), drepanocytes (sickled).
- Color (reflecting concentration of hemoglobin: Normochromic, hypochromic.

Hgb, Hct, MCV, Reticulocyte Count, and Platelets

Hemoglobin Normal values:

- Neonate: 14.5-22.5 g/dl.
- 2 months: 9.0-14.0 g/dl.

Discussion: Carries oxygen and is decreased in anemia and increased in polycythemia.

Hematocrit Normal values:

- Neonate: 48-69%.
- 3 days: 44-75%
- 2 months:28-42%

Discussion: Indicates the proportion of RBCs in a liter of blood (usually about 3 times the hemoglobin number).

Mean corpuscular volume (MCV) Normal values:

- Neonate: 95-121 µm³.
- 0.5-2 years: 70-86 µm³.

Discussion: Indicates the size of RBCs and can differentiate types of anemia. For adults, <80 is microcytic and >100 is macrocytic, but this varies with age.

Reticulocyte count Normal values:

- 0.5-1.5% of total RBCs

Discussion: Measures marrow production and should rise with anemia.

Platelets Normal values:

- 150,000-400,000

Discussion: Are essential for clotting. May increase to >1 million during acute infection or with iron deficiency anemia.

WBCs

Leukocytes are white blood cells (WBCs). Normal total values vary according to age. The differential is the percentage of each type of WBC out of the total. The differential will shift with infection or allergies, but should return to normal values:

Item	Neonate	1 day	2 weeks	1 month
WBCs (X 10³/ mm³)	9.0-30.0	9.4-34.0	5.0-20.0	5.0-19.5.
Myelocytes	0%	0%	0%	0%
Neutrophils (bands)	9.1%	9.2%	5.5%	4.5%
Neutrophils (segs)	52%	52%	34%	30%
Lymphocytes	31%	31%	48%	56%
Monocytes	5.8%	5.8%	8.8%	6.5%
Eosinophils:	2.2%	2.0%	3.1%	2.8%
Basophils	0.6%	0.5%	0.4%	0.5%

<u>Pituitary Hormones</u>

The **anterior pituitary gland (adenohypophysis)** produces hormones that are critical for growth and development:

- **Growth hormone** (GH) promotes growth of bones and muscles and promotes protein synthesis and metabolism of fat but decreases carbohydrate metabolism. Normal values include:
  - Cord blood: 8-40 µg/L. 1 day:5-50 µg/L. 1 week: 5-25 µg/L.
- **Thyroid stimulating hormone** (TSH) stimulates secretion of thyroid hormones. Normal value: Neonates-3 days: < 20 mIU/L.
- **Adrenocorticotropic hormone** (ACTH) stimulates the adrenal glands to produce glucocorticoids, androgens and mineralocorticoids. Abnormalities can result in Cushing's disease or Addison's disease. Normal values:
  - Cord blood: 11-25 pmol/L.
  - Neonate: 2-41 pmol/L.

The **posterior pituitary gland (neurohypophysis)** stores hormones produced by the hypothalamus, critical to renal function. **Antidiuretic hormone** controls the reabsorption of fluids in the kidney tubules. Changes in serum osmolality stimulate or depress ADH secretion, so values vary:

- Serum osmolality 270-280 mOsm/kg: ADH <1.4 pmol/L.
- Serum osmolality 280-285 mOsm/kg: ADH <2.3 pmol/L.
- Serum osmolality 285-290 mOsm/kg: ADH 0.9-4.6 pmol/L.

<u>Thyroid Hormones</u>

The **thyroid gland** produces hormones critical for metabolism and growth. They are amino acids that contain iodine and are stored in the thyroid until needed by the body. The thyroid gland takes iodide from the blood and utilizes it to produce hormones. Thyroid hormone production is controlled by the thyroid stimulating hormone (TSH) produced by the pituitary gland and the thyrotropin-releasing hormone (TRH) produced by the hypothalamus. Together, the thyroid hormones increase metabolic rate and protein and bone turnover. They are necessary for the growth and development of the fetus and infant. Thyroid hormones include:

- **Thyroxine** (T_4) is a weak hormone that maintains the body metabolism in a steady state.
  - Neonate: 10-36 pmol/L.
- **Triiodothyronine** (T_3) is about 5 times stronger than thyroxine and can respond quickly to metabolic needs.
  - All ages: 4.0-7.4 pmol/L.
- **Thyrocalcitonin** is secreted in response to serum calcium levels and reduces the serum level of calcium and phosphate by increasing deposits in bones, aiding ossification and bone development.
  - Male: <19 ng/L.
  - Female: <14 ng/L.

Immunologic Clinical Laboratory Tests

The **immunological** status of infants with HIV positive mothers is assessed in a series of tests performed over the first two years in order to institute treatment and decrease transmission to ≥2%:

- Birth (≥24 hours): ELISA and rapid tests are used to identify those neonates who test positive at birth. Confirmatory testing is done with the neonate's blood (not cord blood), usually using DNA PCR, which is about 99% sensitive by 1 month. RNA PCR may be used for some subtypes of HIV infection.

In the United States, testing is based on identifying mothers with HIV. If the mother's status is not known, then some states require mandatory testing of the infant, but laws vary. Based on positive findings, treatment is begun within 24 hours without waiting for confirmatory test results. Breastfeeding is avoided. Subsequent testing is done at 2, 4, 12, and 18 months.

Genetic Clinical Laboratory Tests

Screening of the newborn to detect genetic diseases varies somewhat from one state to another. Because about 1 in 200 newborns has chromosomal abnormalities, screening is an important tool although many birth defects are not genetic in origin, such as defects caused by maternal alcohol abuse or vitamin deficiency. Screening tests are available for the following:

- Biotinidase deficiency (autosomal recessive).
- Congenital adrenal hyperplasia (autosomal recessive).
- Congenital hearing loss (autosomal recessive, autosomal dominant, or mitochondrial).
- Congenital hypothyroidism (autosomal recessive or autosomal dominant).
- Cystic fibrosis (autosomal recessive).
- Galactosemia (autosomal recessive).
- Homocystinuria (autosomal recessive)
- Maple syrup urine disease (autosomal recessive).
- Medium-chain Acyl-CoA dehydrogenase (autosomal recessive).
- Phenylketonuria (autosomal recessive).
- Sickle cell disease (autosomal recessive).
- Tyrosemia (2 types are autosomal recessive; third type is unclear).

Neonatal Assessment: Diagnostic and Interventional Procedures

Ultrasound/Doppler

Ultrasound is an imaging technique using high-frequency sound waves to create computer images of vessels, tissues, and organs. Newer scans include 2-dimensional **Doppler** readings. Ultrasound is used to view organs, evaluate function, and assess circulation. Infants usually do not require sedation. Ultrasound has the advantages of being portable and not exposing the infant to radiation. Common ultrasounds for the neonate include:

- *Hip*: The ultrasound is done while the hip is placed in various positions to determine placement and ligament integrity.
- *Cranial:* Most images are obtained through the anterior fontanelle with axial images through the temporal bone. The transducer is angled in order to obtain images of various parts of the brain to determine abnormalities.

- **Urinary system:** The ultrasound may be used to determine kidney size and bladder filling.
- **Vascular:** The ultrasound can show vascular abnormalities (usually non-thoracic).
- **Chest**: Ultrasounds are done primarily to assess cardiac function.
- **Abdomen**: Ultrasounds can show abnormalities of abdominal organs, such as intestines, liver, or pancreas.

Computerized Tomography

Computerized tomography (CT) is relatively fast and is used to evaluate neonates who are clinically unstable. A contrast dye may be injected intravenously as blood vessels become brighter with contrast. With the CT, a thin x-ray beam rotates around the patient. The computer then analyzes the data to construct a cross-sectional image, which can be stacked to create a three-dimensional model of organs. The CT scan is more effective than MRI for detecting these factors:

- Calcification.
- Skull lesions.
- Hemorrhage less than 24 hours in duration (hyperacute).

Infants require light sedation to prevent movement, which can blur images, and must be monitored carefully throughout the scan. Infants are at increased risk of excessive radiation exposure from multiple CTs because they receive the same amount of radiation as an adult even though their size is smaller. Parts of the body, such as the genitals, may be shielded to prevent radiation exposure.

Magnetic Resonance Imaging

Magnetic resonance imaging (MRI) is based on the magnetic properties of atoms, so it is safer for infants although they usually require anesthesia, so the infant must be monitored throughout the procedure. Infant earplugs and headphones are used to protect the ears from sound. In some cases, the MRI may be done without anesthesia with the infant sleeping. The infant is kept awake before the MRI and then fed immediately before, swaddled, and rocked or comforted until sleeping. The infant lies on a table that slides into a tunnel-like tube. A small body coil may be placed around the head to send and receive the radio wave pulses for brain scans. The energy from the radio waves is absorbed and then released in a pattern formed by the type of tissue and by certain diseases. Intravenous contrast dye may be administered. Usually several sets of images are taken, each requiring 2-15 minutes so a complete scan may take up to an hour although newer MRIs are faster.

Chest X-Ray

Chest x-ray is one of the leading procedures used to diagnose ailments and illness and in the treatment of respiratory disease in the neonate. The NICU nurse plays an important role in assisting with these x-rays and should understand the different views that may be requested:

- **Anteroposterior view**: In this view the x-ray is placed directly above the infant's chest; the beam passes from front to back. This is the most common view used when assessing a neonate.
- **Cross-table lateral view**: In this view, the infant is placed supine, the x-ray machine points horizontally through the infant the most common time this view is used is to verify line placement.

- *Lateral decubitus view*: The infant is placed with the side that may have a problem up, the arm on that side should be lifted out of the x-ray field. Pneumothorax is usually the suspect when this view is used, by putting the suspected side up, the air will rise and be more evident on the film.

Electrocardiogram

Electrocardiogram (ECG) is a non-invasive, painless, inexpensive way to determine if the myocardium or conduction system is damaged through a graphical representation of the heart's electrical activity over time. Skin electrodes measure electrical potential between different points of the body. The ECG is used to detect and diagnose:

- Arrhythmias.
- Electrolyte imbalances.
- Conduction disorders.
- Myocardial infarction.
- Atrial or ventricular hypertrophy.

The infant should be in supine position and calm. In some cases, this procedure may require sedation. Because of the large size of the heart in a neonate compared to an adult, extra right-sided chest leads (and occasionally left) may be added. Arm leads should be between the shoulder and elbow and leg leads between the hip and knee but proximal to the hip.

ECG Findings

ECG Marking	Seconds/ physiology	Significance
P wave	0.08 - 0.2 Atrial depol.	Enlarged P waves indicate atrial enlargement.
PR interval	0.12 - 0.20 Electricity travels from SA node to ventricles.	AV block = P-R interval >0.2 seconds. 1st degree block = electrical impulse transmits into ventricles.
QRS complex	0.06 - 0.1 Ventricular depolarization.	Enlarged QRS complex = ventricular hypertrophy.
ST segment	0.08 - 0.12 Ventricle depolarizes.	Depression = ischemia. Elevation = hypoxia or MI.
T wave	>QRS Repolarization is slower than depolarization.	Altered by electrolyte abnormalities. Inversion = ischemia or MI.
QT interval	0.2 - 0.4 (Q-Tc <0.44) Ventricular depolarization and repolarization.	Long Q-T = susceptibility to tachyarrhythmias.

Electroencephalogram

The **electroencephalogram** (EEG) records changes of electrical potential in different parts of the brain by electrodes placed on the scalp. EEG is done to diagnose cerebral disease, epilepsy, and CNS effects of various metabolic and systemic disorders. Typically, a standard 10-20 EEG is used, but the number of leads is reduced because of the neonate's small head size, and the EEG tracing is done for about an hour to ensure that both waking and sleeping states are recorded. Physiological leads

- 58 -

(eye-movement monitors, EMG, ECG, respiratory monitors) may be used as well to help to identify the neonate's state. The infant lies in supine position during testing. The infant should be monitored carefully and the time of all movements and behavior that may cause artifacts (sucking, moving, twitching, eye movement) noted. Post-conceptual age (gestational weeks plus weeks after birth) is used during analyses, as there are variations in finding with the neonate's age.

Echocardiogram

An **echocardiogram** is a form of ultrasound used to determine the size, shape, and movement of cardiac structures. High-frequency sound waves are transmitted into the heart by a handheld transducer held against the chest wall; however, images tend to be poor because of interference caused by tissue and bone. Echocardiogram may be done with two-dimensional view Doppler, and some newer equipment can provide a three-dimensional view. Echocardiograms are done to diagnose congenital heart defects, assess ductus arteriosus, monitor pulmonary hypertension, and assess extracardiac abnormalities that may be associated with cardiac abnormalities as well. A more effective method is the **transesophageal echocardiogram** in which a miniaturized transducer is fed through the mouth or nose and down the esophagus, allowing the transducer to be closer to the heart. This is often done during surgical procedures with the child anesthetized.

Voiding Cystourethrogram

Voiding cystourethrogram (VCUG) is a type of x-ray procedure with contrast. Usually, preliminary x-rays are taken and then a catheter is inserted through the urethra into the bladder, which is filled with liquid containing contrast dye, after which the catheter is removed. X-rays are taken as the bladder fills and empties, showing function and reverse flow of urine to ureters and kidneys. The infant is usually swaddled to prevent movement. Discomfort to the infant is minimal, but instillation must be carefully monitored, especially in preterm infants, to avoid rupture or injury to the bladder. The child is generally not sedated or anesthetized because urinating is necessary in order to complete the test. The VCUG should not be done if the infant has an active urinary infection (usual delay after treatment of UTI is 2-4 weeks) and cannot be used to diagnose obstruction from the kidneys to the bladder.

Diagnostic Techniques and Equipment

Bag and Mask Ventilation
Bag and mask ventilation is indicated for persistent apnea or gasping respirations, bradycardia (<100 bpm), and persistent cyanosis unrelieved by free-flowing oxygen.

Flow-inflating bag and mask (Connected to oxygen flow, which inflates bag). Equipment includes:

- Oxygen inlet
- Flow control valve
- Pressure manometer attachment
- Patient outlet for mask attachment

Advantages: Flow-inflating bag and mask ventilation has the ability to deliver anywhere from 21% (room air) to 100% oxygen; any pressure desired can be set. This type of bag and mask also has the ability to maintain positive end-expiratory pressure (PEEP) and CPAP.

Disadvantages: Because this bag must be connected to a gas (oxygen) source to inflate, it can only be used where a gas supply exists. It requires some experience to deliver the desired quantity of air with each breath. The high pressures possible with this type of equipment make over-inflation of

- 59 -

the lungs possible, resulting in pneumothorax. A complete seal is necessary to deliver a tidal volume.

Self-inflating bag and mask (Does not require gas source). Equipment includes:

- Air inlet
- Oxygen inlet
- Patient outlet for mask attachment
- Valve assembly
- Oxygen reservoir
- Pop-off valve
- Pressure manometer attachment

Advantages: Self-inflating bag and mask ventilation is simple to use and does not require much practice or experience to operate. It can be operated anywhere even if no oxygen source is near and can easily deliver a tidal volume.

Disadvantages: These bags usually have a pop-off valve that will open at a pressure set by the manufacturer to prevent over inflation of the lungs. This valve popping off can prevent the ability to deliver enough pressure to ventilate very noncompliant lungs. Another disadvantage is that if 90% or higher oxygen delivery is desired, this equipment must have a reservoir attached to deliver this concentration. The inability to deliver PEEP is also a disadvantage to the self-inflating bag and mask.

Endotracheal Intubation

The difficult airway of neonates makes choosing an age-appropriate **endotracheal tube** (ETT) very important. The formula for estimating ETT sizes: [Age (yr) + 16] / 4 = ETT size (internal diameter in mm). Usually the depth an ETT can be inserted is estimated at 3 times the internal diameter of the ETT (or 12 + age / 2 = length). An acceptable ETT leak is 15-20 cm H_2O pressure. The ETT may be inserted nasally or orally. Premedication (morphine or fentanyl and midazolam) is used to relieve stress on the neonate. Atropine may be given to block vagal response. ETT placement should immediately be verified by auscultation and radiograph, ultrasound, or disposable end-tidal carbon dioxide detectors may be used. Esophageal intubation is indicated if no air exchange is detected bilaterally or if there is air sound over left upper abdomen. The tube may be too high if air sounds are diminished and too low if the right lung is better ventilated than the left.

Umbilical Artery/Vein Catheter

Umbilical catheters may be arterial or venous, depending on primary need:

- Arterial: ABG monitoring, continuous arterial BP monitoring, infusion of parenteral fluids.

Umbilical artery catheter placement: A sterile field must be maintained, so the infant's arms and legs are restrained to prevent contamination. The infant's temperature must be monitored and maintained at 36-37 °C (by placing on radiant heater or in heated incubator). The child is placed in supine position and the umbilical cord and surrounding skin cleansed with povidone iodine and then alcohol or sterile water. For infants <1250 g a 3.5 Fr. catheter is used, and for those >1250 g, 5 Fr. catheter. After sterile draping, iris forceps are used to dilate one of the arteries and the catheter inserted. If resistance is felt at the umbilical cord tie, it may need to be loosened. The inserted length correlates to the infant's length (using chart), traveling inferiorly and then superiorly (leg loop). Blood should be aspirated and extremities observed for circulatory compromise. Radiograph verifies correct placement.

Umbilical catheters may be inserted into the umbilical vein. This is easy to identify as there is only one, it is larger than the arteries, and it is usually open and does not require dilation. Indications for using the umbilical vein include:

- Venous: Exchange transfusions, CVP monitoring, and emergency administration of fluids.

Umbilical vein catheter placement: Catheter size is 3.5 Fr. for ELBW infants or 5 Fr. (most common). Length of placement is estimated by measuring the length from the umbilicus to the sternal notch and multiplying this number by 0.6. The procedure for insertion is similar to that for the umbilical artery, but insertion is usually easier. The catheter should be in the inferior vena cava, above the diaphragm but below right atrium. Placement should be verified by echocardiography, as radiograph may not provide adequate visualization.

Peripheral Catheterization

Peripheral catheterization of the radial artery (most common) may be done instead of the umbilical artery to monitor blood gases and blood pressure. A 22-24-gauge IV catheter with stylet is used after ulnar collateral flow is assessed in the hand by compressing the radial and ulnar arteries and then releasing the ulnar artery and ensuring that the entire hand flushes. The wrist is extended and the hand secured using an appropriately-sized arm board for support. Transillumination may be used to facilitate passing the cannula into the artery. Once the artery is entered, the stylet is removed and the catheter advanced. If there is no blood return, the catheter is slightly withdrawn until blood flows and then advanced. Heparinized saline solution is instilled into the catheter to prevent thrombus formation. For exchange transfusions, both the radial artery and a superficial vein are catheterized, and blood is withdrawn from the arterial catheter and new blood infused through the venous catheter at the rate of 5 mL/kg/min.

Chest Tube Insertion/Removal

Chest tubes are inserted in the neonate to treat pneumothorax causing cardiac or respiratory compromise or pleural effusion. Transillumination may be used to identify the area of pneumothorax but chest x-ray is more accurate. An 8-12 Fr. chest tube is placed anteriorly for collections of air and posteriorly/laterally for fluid. The infant is supine with the arm at 90° on the insertion side. Insertion sites:

- Anterior: Mid-clavicular line, 2nd or 3rd intercostal space.
- Posterior/lateral: Anterior axillary line, 4th, 5th, or 6th intercostal space.

Lidocaine is instilled and an incision made over the rib below the target intercostal space. The tissue is spread and the pleura punctured above the rib with a hemostat, expelling air. The chest tube is inserted 2-3cm in preterm and 3-4cm in full term infants. The pursestring suture is tightened and the chest tube attached to a 2-3 bottle or Pleur-Evac underwater seal system. X-ray confirms placement. Chest tube is removed quickly and pressure dressing applied if no bubbling for 24 hours and radiograph clear.

Pleur-Evac System for Chest Tube

A chest tube is attached to a three-chamber system called a **Pleur-Evac.** As the name indicates, there are three separate chambers in this collection system:

- The first chamber is the ***collection chamber***. This chamber is where the air and/or fluid that is being drained from the pleural space as a result of a pulmonary air leak. Bubbling in this chamber is the result of air being pumped out of the pleural space and is expected.

- 61 -

- The second chamber is the ***water seal chamber***; this chamber is where the water in an amount prescribed by the physician is placed to create the vacuum necessary to pull the fluid and/or air out of the pleural space. The amount of water placed in this chamber affects the amount of pressure and should be carefully monitored to make sure it remains at the ordered level.
- The third chamber is the ***suction chamber***, which is responsible for the suction that creates the pressure removing the air from the pleural space.

Needle Aspiration

Neonates receiving bag and mask ventilation or mechanical ventilation risk developing a pneumothorax. Signs of pneumothorax include: Rapid deterioration; poor oxygenation; tachypnea; increased work of breathing; impaired circulation; unequal air entry into lungs; displaced apical heartbeat; and increased transillumination on the affected side. A chest x-ray confirms the diagnosis if the neonate's clinical status allows it. Air is removed via **needle aspiration:**

Equipment	Procedure
Oral sucrose	Give oral sucrose.
1% lidocaine	Place infant in supine position.
Fentanyl	Swab second and third intercostal spaces in midclavicular line with
21 gauge butterfly needle	alcohol.
10 ml syringe	Infiltrate site with 1% lidocaine 0.5 ml to 1 ml.
3-way stopcock attached	Drape insertion site.
to the syringe	Give 250 mcg fentanyl over 2-3 minutes IV.
70% isopropyl alcohol	Insert needle directly into second or third intercostal space in mid-
swab	clavicular line until air is aspirated into syringe.
Sterile gloves	Expel air through stopcock.

Spinal/Lumbar Tap

A **lumbar/spinal tap** is done to obtain cerebrospinal fluid (CSF) for diagnosis of CNS disorder, to monitor treatment, to relieve pressure, and to provide intrathecal medications. The infant is positioned in either the sitting or lateral decubitus position with the head and legs flexed, ensuring that the airway is patent. The insertion site should be identified (L4-L5 interspace). The skin is prepped and infant draped and lidocaine administered. The needle is inserted slowly, aiming toward the umbilicus, and the stylet is removed frequently to check for CSF because the "pop" that is felt with older children and adults is not felt with neonates. Once fluid flows, about 1 mL should be collected in 4 separate specimen tubes for laboratory examination. Once the specimens are collected or adequate fluid has drained, the stylet is replaced, the needle removed, and a pressure dressing applied. The child is placed in supine position.

Suprapubic Bladder Aspiration

Suprapubic bladder aspiration is used to obtain uncontaminated urine for culture. A 21-22 gauge one-inch needle with a 3-5 mL syringe is used. A sterile container should be available. The infant should not have urinated in the hour before the procedure. The urine is placed supine and legs abducted (frog leg) and held in place by an assistant. The puncture site is 1-2cm superior to the pubic symphysis, midline. After the site is cleaned with antiseptic, the needle is inserted at an angle of 90°. The syringe is aspirated while the needle is advanced until the point that urine aspirates. The needle must not advance more than 1 inch because it could puncture the posterior wall of the bladder. The syringe is filled, the needle removed quickly, and a pressure dressing applied. The

- 62 -

urine is instilled into the sterile container. Slight bleeding is common, but excessive bleeding usually relates to a bleeding disorder. The bowel may be perforated if the needle is inserted incorrectly.

PICC Lines

Percutaneously inserted central catheters (PICC) are used for extended intravenous access or those with limited access, and as a transition from umbilical catheters. Insertion sites include the scalp, axilla, and brachial cephalic saphenous veins. The catheter insertion length is measured:

- Hand/arm: Insertion site to axilla and to 1 cm above nipple line.
- Scalp: Insertion site to 1 cm above nipple line.
- Leg: Insertion site to 1 cm above umbilicus.

Topical (EMLA) or local anesthetic is used and the infant's temperature maintained at 36-37°C. Limbs are restrained to prevent contamination of sterile field. If catheter is inserted in the hand or arm, the infant's head is turned toward insertion site to partially occlude the jugular vein and reduce risk of catheter entering the jugular. After insertion above the waist, the catheter should be in the superior vena cava above the right atrium. PICC lines in lower extremities should lie in the inferior vena cava below the right atrium. AP and lateral radiographs, ultrasound, or echocardiogram verify correct placement.

Capillary Blood Sampling

Neonatal **capillary blood sampling** is a common procedure used to acquire small samples of blood for testing of glucose and drug levels, blood gases, electrolytes, urea, blood counts, and other screening tests. If done incorrectly, it can cause pain, trauma, and nerve damage. The lancet should be ≥2.4mm deep. The baby should be supine. The NNP grasps the foot with one hand holding the ankle with the thumb and index finger and supporting the leg with the other fingers. The infant's heel (bottom, lateral aspect only to avoid nerves in the middle of the foot) should be cleansed thoroughly with water (not alcohol) and air-dried. The skin of the heel should be held tense until after the puncture, and then it is relaxed and the heel lightly compressed to express a drop of blood, which is collected in a capillary tube. Relaxing the pressure and then compressing again will "milk" additional drops. Pressure is applied to the puncture site until bleeding stops and then a dressing is applied.

Tracheostomy Management

A **tracheostomy** in the neonate is done in emergent situations, such as upper airway obstruction or abnormalities, and elective situations, such as for prolonged ventilation or subglottic stenosis related to endotracheal intubation. The tracheostomy tube should extend to 1 cm superior to the carina. Because of small size (2.5-3cm inner diameter), neonatal tracheostomy tubes have no inner cannula and are usually not cuffed. Humidity must be provided by attaching the tracheostomy to a warmed humidified air source or use of heat-moisture exchangers. Suctioning, to maintain patency is done every 4 hours with the suction catheter extending slightly below (3-5 mm) the tracheostomy tube, and the suctioning length should be prominently posted. There is no consensus on the use of saline instillation during suctioning. Tubes should be changed regularly, usually at least once weekly. Skin about the stoma should be inspected twice daily and drainage cleansed with saline or hydrogen peroxide/saline (if crusting). In some cases, a thin gauze or hydrocolloid dressing may be placed under the flanges.

Cardiopulmonary Monitoring

Cardiopulmonary monitoring includes electrocardiogram (ECG) and respiratory sensors. Usually 3 chest ECG leads that record the electrical activity of the heart and sense respiratory movement are placed, and the patterns are recorded on a visual screen. Many computerized monitors have memory capability so that data can be analyzed out of real time. They can also be set to record certain events, such as periods of apnea. Alarm thresholds are set, so that an alarm indicates dangerous changes. Apnea alarms should be both visual and auditory. False alarms may occur and should be thoroughly evaluated for cause, such as loose leads or movement. Home monitors include records of compliance so that a review of data shows the time the monitor was actually in use. Home monitors are used for infants at risk for SIDS. Because of interference problems that might provide inaccurate readings, monitors should never be used as a sole evaluation of cardiopulmonary status. Observation and examination must be used to verify the infant's condition.

Non-Invasive Monitoring of Infant on Oxygen

Non-invasive **monitoring** of the neonate receiving **oxygen** includes:

- **Heart rate monitor**: Should show beats per minute as well as a visual depiction of the heart rhythm.
- **Respiratory monitor**: Should show respiratory rate as well as a visual wave showing the pattern of breathing. Alarms should be turned on for apnea and tachypnea.
- **Blood pressure monitor**: Peripheral cuff type monitoring, this does not need to be continuous but needs to be done at regular intervals determined by the physician or practitioner.
- **Pulse oximetry:** Should be a continuous monitoring with alarms set for ordered lower limits.
- **Oxygen analyzer:** Shows the oxygen level being delivered to the neonate.

Non-Invasive Transcutaneous O_2/CO_2 Monitoring

Non-invasive **transcutaneous O2/CO2 monitoring** includes skin oxygen tension ($TCPO_2$) and carbon dioxide tension ($TCPCO_2$). One or two leads are placed on the infant's skin over any part of the body that allows good contact. O_2 and CO_2 diffuse through the skin and monitors provide a digital display. If right-to-left shunting is suspected, then leads are usually placed on right shoulder and lower abdomen or leg (above and below the ductus arteriosus). The electrodes are calibrated (usually every 4 hours to ensure accuracy), and then heat (43-44° C) the underlying skin, but they must be left in place for 15-minutes after calibration to ensure adequate heating of the skin. The electrodes can cause erythema (first-degree burns), so they should be repositioned every 2-4 hours. The electrodes should not be placed beneath the infant because the pressure against it can impede circulation.

End-Tidal CO_2 Monitors

End-tidal CO_2 monitors are used to confirm correct placement of endotracheal tubes during intubation and to ensure adequate oxygenation. Both sidestream analysis with a double lumen ETT and mainstream analysis within the ventilator circuit are used. Clinical assessment alone is not adequate:

- **Capnography** is attached to the ETT and provides a waveform graph, showing the varying concentrations of CO2 in real time throughout each ventilation (with increased CO2 on expiration) and can indicate changes in respiratory status.

A typical waveform rises with expiration (indicating CO2 level), plateaus, and then falls with inspiration (and intake of oxygen). Changes in the height or shape of the waveform can indicate respiratory compromise. Pressure of end-tidal CO_2 (PETCO$_2$) is useful for neonates with normal lung function or in premature infants with mild-moderate lung disease, but results may be inaccurate if there is a large alveolar-arterial gradient.

Pulse Oximetry

Pulse oximetry is a monitoring of the saturation level of the hemoglobin in the blood. For example, a reading of 98% indicates that, of the hemoglobin available, 98% of it is bound to oxygen or saturated with oxygen. This machine uses infrared light to read the hemoglobin. One of the main things that can affect the accuracy of this reading is the perfusion status of the neonate. If the infant is suffering from a condition that results in poor perfusion (hypovolemia, hypotension, etc.), the pulse oximetry reading will be inaccurate as the machine will have difficulty reading the blood. Phototherapy as used for jaundice will also cause inaccurate readings because it is a light as is the tool used in pulse oximetry. The third factor that can result in low pulse oximetry readings is use of Dopamine. Dopamine is a potent vasoconstricting drug. If the veins are constricted, blood flow is affected, causing problems reading the blood for oxygen levels.

Invasive Blood Gas Monitoring

- **Arterial blood gas (ABG)** is the most informative measurement of blood gas status. If an infant has an umbilical artery catheter, it is easily obtained by aspirating 1-2 mL of blood.
- **Venous blood gas (VBG)** is easier to obtain if an arterial catheter is not in place. In order to compare the values in the VBG with an ABG, make the following calculations:
  - Add .05 to the pH of the VBG.
  - Subtract 5-10 mm/Hg from the PCO$_2$ of the VBG.
- **Capillary Blood Gas (CBG)** can be obtained with a heel stick, without a venous or arterial line, but the values obtained in a CBG are the least accurate and are rarely useful. The oxygen status of the neonate (reflected in the PO$_2$) can be estimated by clinical evaluation of the neonate and a noninvasive pulse oximeter reading.

Phototherapy

Phototherapy is commonly used to treat hyperbilirubinemia and jaundice when the total serum bilirubin (TSB) indicates the infant is at risk. Phototherapy is a treatment in which the infant is placed under special lights that decrease the bilirubin levels in the blood. The lights usually consist of one tungsten halogen lamp or 4-8 white or blue fluorescent lights and a Plexiglas® shield. The infant is placed under these lights with a protective mask covering the eyes to prevent retinal toxicity. The lights should be 15-20 cm above the infant. The lights convert bilirubin into a water-soluble compound that can be excreted by the liver into bile and eventually into the infant's stool. The success of phototherapy is directly related to the quantity of body surface area that is exposed to the lights, so the infant is clad only in a diaper to expose the most skin to the light as possible.

Indwelling Catheters—Broviac®

Broviac® catheters are large-bore silastic indwelling catheters that may be surgically (cutdown) or needle inserted if percutaneous insertion is not possible. The most common sites for insertion are the internal or external jugular vein and the common facial vein. Broviac® catheters are most commonly used if long-term access (months, years) is required, such as for parenteral nutrition or medications. A Broviac® catheter is tunneled subcutaneously and exits through the anterior chest. Placement is confirmed with radiograph. The Broviac® catheter is cuffed at the exit point to decrease infection, but the catheter still poses a high risk of infection, especially with frequent administration of parenteral nutrition. Complications include pneumothorax, hemothorax, air embolism, misplacement or occlusion of catheter. The catheter must be secured as it is easily dislodged, so length and positioning should be carefully documented and the catheter checked frequently. The catheter is flushed with heparin to maintain patency and prevent thrombus formation.

Incubators

The goal of placing an infant in an **incubator** is to provide a neutral thermal environment (NTE) that places minimal stress on the infant. Most incubators are rigid, box-like structures like an Isolette, in which an infant is kept in a controlled environment to receive medical care. The infant is allowed to grow and mature here before being transitioned to the more "uncontrolled" environment of an open crib. Features that incubators possess that enhance the production of a NTE include a heater, a fan to circulate warmed air, and a humidity control. They also usually have a way to increase the oxygen content of the environment and ports to allow for nursing care without removing the infant. A servo-control is used in conjunction with a temperature-sensing thermistor that is attached to the infant to help regulate the infant's temperature within a set range. Some incubators may have double walls that lessen radiant heat loss. Infants who are in need of close monitoring are not placed in an incubator, but instead are placed under a radiant warmer with minimal covering. This allows the nurse to monitor the infant's skin color and breathing patterns more closely.

Radiant Warmers

Radiant warmers are devices that provide overhead heat directly to the infant. Radiant heaters provide an area for direct observation and free access to the infant, which is very useful in the initial evaluation and resuscitation (if necessary) of the newborn, or for procedures such as intubation or line placement. Radiant heat devices work best if the room temperature is kept above 25°C. Two problems related to radiant warmers include:

- Promote dehydration if an infant is placed under them for a prolonged amount of time, especially if the infant is premature.
- Risk overheating the infant or cause first-degree burns.

Temperature sensors must be appropriately placed and the infant's temperature monitored frequently to ensure the infant is not being over or under heated.

Non-Invasive Positive Pressure Ventilators

Non-invasive positive pressure ventilators provide air through a tight-fitting nasal or facemask, usually pressure cycled, avoiding the need for intubation and reducing the danger of hospital-acquired infection and mortality rates. It can be used for acute respiratory failure and pulmonary edema. There are 2 types of non-invasive positive pressure ventilators:

- *CPAP (Continuous positive airway pressure)* provides a steady stream of pressurized air throughout both inspiration and expiration. CPAP improves breathing by decreasing preload and afterload for patients with congestive heart failure. It reduces the effort required for breathing and improves compliance of the lung.
- *Bi-PAP (Bi-level positive airway pressure)* provides a steady stream of pressurized air as CPAP but it senses inspiratory effort and increases pressure during inspiration. Bi-PAP pressures for inspiration and expiration can be set independently. Machines can be programmed with a backup rate to ensure a set number of respirations per minute.

Positive Pressure Ventilators

Positive pressure ventilators assist respiration by applying pressure directly to the airway, inflating the lungs, forcing expansion of the alveoli, and facilitating gas exchange. Generally, endotracheal intubation or tracheostomy is necessary to maintain positive pressure ventilation. There are 3 basic kinds of positive pressure ventilators:

- ***Pressure cycled:*** This type of ventilation is usually used for short-term treatment in adolescents or adults. The IPPB machine is the most common type. This delivers a flow of air to a preset pressure and then cycles off. Airway resistance or changes in compliance can affect volume of air and may compromise ventilation.
- ***Time cycled:*** This type of ventilation regulates the volume of air the infant receives by controlling the length of inspiration and the flow rate. This type of ventilator is used almost exclusively for neonates and infants.
- ***Volume cycled:*** This type of ventilation provides a preset flow of pressurized air during inspiration and then cycles off and allows passive expiration, providing a fairly consistent volume of air.

Circumcision

Circumcision is becoming less common, with only about 58% of male infants now circumcised in the United States. Some people still choose circumcision for religious or personal reasons. While, at one time, infants were not thought to experience pain, it is now clear that they do, so circumcision is done under anesthesia of some type, usually a topical anesthetic, dorsal penile nerve block, or subcutaneous ring block. Techniques include the use of the Gomco clamp, the Mogen clam, the Plastibell clamp, or a scalpel alone. Typically, the end of the foreskin is swollen and red after circumcision, and some bleeding may persist for 24 hours. Contraindications include bleeding disorders and genital abnormalities. Complications include infection, persistent bleeding, incomplete removal, and injury to the glans or penis, meatal stenosis, necrosis, urethrocutaneous fistula, and phimosis.

Care includes:

- Changing the diaper immediately because urine may cause pain to the open tissue.
- Cleansing the area gently with water and pat dry, apply petrolatum gauze about the site for 24 hours and then petrolatum jelly until healed.
- Avoiding the use of soap or commercial cleansing products, such as baby wipes, until the circumcision heals.

Family Integration

Decreasing Family Stress

Having a neonate admitted to the neonatal intensive care unit is a very stressful event for a family because it interrupts family interactions and the bonding process that occurs when a neonate goes home to spend time with family members. Steps to decrease **family stress** and encourage bonding between the neonate, mother, and family include:

- Have facilities available for families to stay close to their infant to encourage bonding.
- Maintain a play area for siblings so they are not isolated from parents.
- Permit liberal visiting times for family members.

- If it is known before birth that the infant will require critical care, let the family visit the unit and ask questions.
- Give the family contact information for support groups comprised of other parents who have children with similar illnesses.
- Encourage hands-on parental care, including kangaroo care, by both parents.

Sibling Responses/Interventions

Siblings should be included, and parents are encouraged to bring them to visit and interact, as much as possible, with the neonate. If the neonate has abnormalities, this may cause stress to the siblings. Younger children may be hostile and older children ashamed. They may feel guilty about their responses, and they may feel neglected as parents go through the stages of grief and are unable to provide the support that the siblings need. In some cases, parents may express their concern by focusing their anxiety on one of the siblings, becoming hypercritical. In these cases, staff may need to intervene by discussing observations with the parents and encouraging other family members to provide support to the siblings. Parents' groups that involve the entire family can be very helpful. Whenever possible, children should be included in education and demonstrations and encouraged to ask questions. Age-appropriate books and other materials that explain medical conditions and treatments should be available for siblings.

Barriers to Parent Infant Interaction

There are many barriers to **parent-infant interaction**, especially with preterm infants or those with genetic disabilities/birth defects that require prolonged hospitalization or treatment. Barriers include:

- *Physical separation:* When the infant cannot be held or fed, when the child is transported to a different facility outside of the area, or when the mother is discharged and the infant remains hospitalized, this prevents attachment.
- *Lack of clear understanding of handicaps/developmental problems:* Lack of infant response is sometimes interpreted as rejection, and parents may be frightened by abnormalities.
- *Attitude of medical staff:* Negative attitudes may cause the parent to grieve rather than attach to the child. Staff members need to encourage the parents to become involved in the child's care and provide stimulation. Staff often needs to demonstrate care to parents, who may be intimidated by the infant's condition and medical needs.
- *Environmental overload:* The equipment (alarms, ventilators, monitors) and environmental constraints (no chairs) may overwhelm parents.

Stages of Grief

Grief is a normal response to the death or severe illness/abnormality of an infant or fetus. How a person deals with grief is very personal, and each person will grieve differently. Elisabeth Kubler-Ross identified **five stages of grief** in *On Death and Dying* (1969). A person may not go through each stage but usually goes through two of the five stages:

- *Denial*: The parents may be resistive to information and unable to accept that a child is dying/impaired or believe that the child is not theirs. They may act stunned, immobile, or detached and may be unable to respond appropriately or remember what's said, often repeatedly asking the same questions.

- *Anger*: As reality becomes clear, parents may react with pronounced anger, directed inward or outward. Women, especially, may blame themselves and self-anger may lead to severe depression and guilt, assuming they are to blame because of some action before or during pregnancy. Outward anger, more common in men, may be expressed as overt hostility.
- *Bargaining*: This involves if-then thinking (often directed at a deity): "If I go to church every way, then God will prevent this." Parents may change doctors, trying to change the outcome.
- *Depression*: As the parents begin to accept the loss, they may become depressed, feeling no one understands and overwhelmed with sadness. They may be tearful or crying and may withdraw or ask to be left alone.
- *Acceptance*: This final stage represents a form of resolution and often occurs outside of the medical environment after months. Parents are able to resume their normal activities and lose the constant preoccupation with their child. They are able to think of the child without severe pain. With a disabled child, acceptance may be delayed because of daily challenges and reminders.

Types of Grief

Anticipatory grief occurs when a child is diagnosed with a terminal illness. The parent begins to mourn over the loss of the child before he or she expires.

Incongruent grief occurs when the mother and the father are "out of synch" in their grieving process, stressing their relationship. It may be due to the differences in how men and women grieve, or it may be because the woman typically bonds with the infant during the pregnancy, while the father bonds after the child is born.

Delayed grief occurs when the grieving process is postponed months to years after the loss of a child. Initially, the parent may not be able to grieve appropriately, because of an inability to cope, or the pressing need to care for other family members.

Grief (Gender Differences)

When faced with the death of a child, **men and women** generally grieve differently:

- Women are often more expressive about their loss and more emotional. They are more likely to look for support from others. Men often grieve in a more solitary and cognitive manner. They are generally more oriented to fact gathering or problem-solving.
- The bond that develops between a pregnant woman and the developing fetus is unique and generally very intense. The father often forms a stronger bond after the birth of the child.

When one parent does not grieve in the same fashion as the other (incongruent grieving) this may be a source of conflict in their marriage. How a person acts on the outside is not always a true indicator of how a person is feeling on the inside.

Factors That Influence a Grieving Family

The emotions that individuals and families experience with the loss of an infant are varied and dependent on many **factors**, including:

- *Cultural influences*: Different cultures have their own practices and beliefs concerning death and dying, and varying rituals and ceremonies for processing loss.
- *Family system*: The family's composition, the roles of various members, and economic circumstances affect its expression of grief. A large family with extended community support processes grief differently than a single mother living far from home.
- *Siblings*: The impact of the loss on other children in the family must be considered rather than concentrating on the parents alone.
- *History of loss*: Many diseases have a genetic component, and this may not be the first child the family has lost.

Discharge Planning

Discharge Requirements

In the past, **discharge requirements** included weight or post conceptual weight requirements. Current requirements are instead based on physiological and functional readiness. Hospitals vary, but requirements generally include:

- All medical or surgical problems that require hospitalization are resolved
- The infant is feeding appropriately, as evidenced by:
  - Primary caregiver feeding the infant with the prescribed method (gavage, gastrostomy, or special positioning).
  - Weight gain of 15-30 grams per day over several days.
  - Feeds accomplished without respiratory difficulty.
- Temperature stability is maintained in an open crib.
- Parents are trained appropriately concerning administration of medications, CPR, and proper use of car seat.
- Infant has passed all pre-discharge tests:
  - Hearing screening.
  - Other tests as needed (anemia, ROP exams, sleep study, head ultrasound).
- Age appropriate immunizations were administered.
- Discharge environment has been evaluated.
- Appropriate post discharge follow-up appointments are scheduled with specialists and the primary care physician.

Discharge Planning for the Preterm Infant

Family involvement and education are vital for successful **discharge of the premature infant** to ensure proper care. Bringing home a premature infant or one who has special needs is a daunting task for any parent. Before discharge, the following should be done:

- Educate the parents or guardian about appropriate caring methods.
- Explain how to interpret the infant's cues concerning his needs and how to respond appropriately.

- Point out the different states of alertness during their infant's sleep and wake cycles. Identify the appropriate times and methods for infant interaction.
- Coach the parents to ensure they perform each skill correctly and retain it. Observe interaction between the infant and parents in the nursery to help ensure continued wellness of the infant after discharge.
- Encourage kangaroo care immediately after birth for stable newborns because it is an excellent method to foster bonding between the neonate and the mother. For neonates who require resuscitation and medical intervention, delay kangaroo care until the neonate is stable.
- If the parents are not ready, contact Social Work for follow-up.

Anticipatory Guidance for an Infants

Infants with Congenital Rubella Syndrome

Infants who have been diagnosed as having **congenital rubella syndrome** will secrete this active virus in their urine and stool for many years after birth. This requires that parents be extensively taught about the risk their infant could pose to pregnant women who are not immune to rubella or who do not know their status. The mother of an infant with this disorder should have a titer drawn to ensure that they are shown as immune so as to prevent future pregnancies from being affected. The parents need to be taught that they have a responsibility to protect others from exposure but to make sure that in the process they are not treating the infant in such a way so as to completely isolate him from the outside world.

Infants Requiring Home Cardiorespiratory Monitors

Some infants may be discharged from the NICU on **cardiorespiratory monitors**. These monitors have been shown to be successful in preventing death from apnea for certain infants. These monitors are NOT indicated for the prevention of SIDS in an otherwise healthy newborn. The following events are indications that an infant may be sent home on monitors:

- Infant who has apnea of prematurity that has had all other causes of apnea ruled out.
- Infant who survived an apparent life-threatening event (ALTE) and that event was apnea, cyanosis, choking or gagging.
- Infant who has had two or more siblings who have died from SIDS
- Infant with a tracheostomy.

Parents/caregivers must have a clear understanding of the reasons for the monitors and how to apply, remove, and care for them. They should have hospital practice and should demonstrate their skills before discharge of the infants.

Infants Exposed to Substances of Abuse While *in Utero*

Infants exposed to perinatal drugs of abuse require a multidisciplinary team approach when preparing for discharge. These high-risk infants may still be dealing with physical withdrawal symptoms. They have possible developmental delays. They may return to a toxic home (marijuana grow-op, methamphetamine lab, crack house, or bordello). Ensure that:

- A case manager is assigned to all infants to coordinate the discharge process.
- Postpartum length of stay is flexible, as the infant may not display symptoms of withdrawal until 7 days of age.
- The mother is allowed to room-in to facilitate special teaching concerning withdrawal symptoms and to strengthen the infant-maternal bonding process.

- 71 -

- A public health nurse or protective social worker is scheduled to perform a home evaluation within one week of discharge.
- Mothers (and fathers) who are not already enrolled in a drug abuse treatment program are referred to an appropriate program.

Infants with Cardiac Disorder

Parents caring for an **infant with a cardiac disorder** should be taught to call the physician if their infants exhibit any of the following symptoms:

- Poor feeding that lasts more than a couple of days.
- Sweating or grunting while feeding (any signs that feeding is extra work or tiring them out).
- Vomiting the majority of what is eaten in a 12-24-hour period of time.
- Breathing that is faster than normal or that looks or sounds labored and lasts for several hours.
- A significant and noticeable decrease in the activity level of the infant.
- Any weight loss or failure to gain weight for a significant period of time.
- A change in skin or perioral color (cyanosis).
- A higher than normal incidence of respiratory type illnesses (cold, croup, etc.).

These instructions should be written down for the parents to take home and refer to, as one cannot rely on the memory of already stressed parents for something this important.

Follow-Up Screening from Neonate to Childhood

Many **screening procedures** are available; including extensive laboratory testing that may be indicated if there is cause for concern that an infant may have a disorder. However, some basic screening should be done for all infants and children:

- *Genetic disorders:* Screening is usually done at birth according to state guidelines, and then may be indicated if there is concern that a child has a disorder that requires treatment.
- *Hearing:* Testing is usually done with newborns between 3-8 years and then every 2-3 years until age 18.
- *Height and weight:* These are monitored monthly during the first year and then at least yearly until age 18 to determine if the child's development is within the normal range.
- *Vision:* This is screened at birth, at 3-4 years, and periodically between 5-18. Vision problems may become obvious when the child enters school and can't see the board or has trouble reading.
- *Fasting blood sugar:* Done every 2 years for those at risk.
- *Head circumference:* Measurement is done at birth, 1 year, and 2 years.
- *Blood pressure:* This is usually checked during infancy (6-12 months) and then periodically throughout childhood.
- *Dental screening:* Bottle fed babies may require earlier screening as they often fall asleep with the bottle in their mouths, leading to infant caries. Dental screening is done periodically throughout childhood, especially after the new teeth come in to evaluate for malocclusion or other problems.
- *Alcohol/drug use:* Neonates are screened for parental abuse. Screening of use may be done periodically for children between 11-18 years, especially if they are at risk.

- *Developmental screening:* There are a number of screening tests that are available and can be used if a child appears to have a developmental delay or abnormality. Screening tests must be age-appropriate. The tests are not diagnostic, but can help to confirm developmental abnormalities. Tests may assess motor skills, language, and cognitive ability.

Universal Hearing Screening Prior to Discharge

Universal hearing screening is recommended by the AAP for all newborns. Hearing loss in neonates may occur because of genetic abnormalities, *in utero* infections with cytomegalovirus or rubella, meningitis, craniofacial abnormalities, or Usher's syndrome. Admission to the NICU for longer than two days increases the likelihood of hearing loss by 10-fold, so all newborns should be screened for hearing loss — not just those with risk factors — prior to discharge. Undiagnosed hearing loss results in severe language and developmental delay. Identification and early intervention during the critical time period of language development decreases the morbidity associated with neonatal hearing loss. Reasons for screening include:

- An easy-to-use test is available with high degrees of sensitivity and specificity.
- Hearing loss is otherwise difficult to detect until language milestones have been missed
- Interventions are available to correct conditions.
- Early intervention results in improved outcome.
- The screening process can be performed in a cost-effective manner.

General Management

Thermoregulation

Heat Transfer Mechanisms

There are four **heat transfer mechanisms** to consider when caring for a neonate, especially a premature one: conduction, convection, radiation, and evaporation. Mechanisms include:

- **Conduction**: The transfer of heat between solid objects of different temperatures in contact with each other. Heat is transferred from the body of the infant to a cold surface they may come into contact with, such as a scale. Care should be taken to make sure the scales are warmed before use. Conduction can also be used to warm the infant by placing a warmed blanket next to the skin to conduct the warmth to the infant.
- **Convection**: The transfer of heat through air currents to the air moving around and across an infant's body. Incubators use convection of warm air being pumped into the incubator to keep an infant warm. Heat can be lost this way if a cool draft is allowed to be near the infant.

Radiation and evaporation are two additional heat transfer mechanisms:

- **Radiation**: Heat transferred between two objects not in contact with each other. This is the transfer of heat through emission of infrared rays. Radiant warming beds use this mechanism to warm the infant. Heat loss occurs when an infant is in an incubator and the walls of the incubator are cooler than body temperature. The neonate in an incubator with this situation will lose body heat through radiation from his body to the cooler walls despite the warm air being pumped in.
- **Evaporation**: Loss of heat occurring when moisture evaporates from the surface of the skin. Evaporation is the result of conversion of liquid into a vapor and is a major concern at birth, as a wet infant can experience a 3-degree drop in body temperature in only about 10 minutes. Thus, drying and replacing wet linens with warm and dry ones is critical at birth.

Heat Loss in Preterm Infants

Preterm infants have not yet developed many of the features that full-term infants use to help protect them from heat loss. The characteristics that make premature infants especially vulnerable to cold stress include:

- Larger surface area to body mass ratio that allows for quicker transfer of body heat to the environment.
- Decreased amounts of subcutaneous fat that provides insulation from heat loss.
- Decreased amounts of brown fat used for non-shivering thermogenesis.
- Immature skin that is not completely keratinized is more permeable to evaporative water and heat loss.
- Inability to flex the body to conserve heat.
- Limited control of skin blood flow mechanisms that conserve heat.

Evaporative Heat Loss and Humidity

Evaporative heat loss occurs when moisture vaporizes from the skin of an infant. In infants born younger than 31 weeks gestation, evaporative heat loss is greatly enhanced by the poor keratinization of the infant's skin. Poor keratinization makes skin highly permeable, which

- 74 -

promotes both fluid and heat loss. This permeability decreases 7-10 days after birth. The amount of evaporation is dependent on the relative humidity of the environment. The more **humid the environment**, the more that evaporation and its associated heat loss are suppressed. A dry environment promotes evaporative heat and fluid loss through the skin. An incubator with humidity controls should be used for infants who are vulnerable to evaporative heat loss. Infants prone to temperature instability should be kept in a highly humid environment.

Minimizing Heat Loss

At delivery, **minimize heat loss** while evaluating the newborn by following these steps:

- Dry the infant thoroughly (including hair) to minimize evaporative heat loss, and remove wet towels.
- Place a cap on the infant's head, as the head is the most significant area of heat loss.
- When the infant is to be weighed, cover the scales with a warm cloth to minimize conductive heat loss.
- Place infant in a warm environment such as:
  o Skin-to-skin contact with mother, and cover them with a warm blanket.
  o Bundled in warm blankets and given to mother to hold.
  o Underneath a preheated warmer for further evaluation or resuscitation.

Minimizing heat loss is especially important if the newborn is premature or has intrauterine growth restriction, but full-term newborns also suffer if they become chilled.

Non-Shivering Thermogenesis (NST)

Non-shivering thermogenesis (NST) is the major route of rapid increase of body temperature in response to cold stress in the term neonate. NST is the oxidation of brown fat to create heat. Brown adipose tissue contains a high concentration of stored triglycerides, a rich capillary network, and is controlled by the sympathetic nervous system. Brown fat cells have a rich supply of mitochondria that are unique, in that when fat is metabolized ATP is not produced, but instead heat is created. Temperature regulation is controlled by the posterior hypothalamus. When a cold body temperature is detected, the posterior hypothalamus responds by triggering the adrenal glands to release norepinephrine and the pituitary gland to release thyroxine. Both norepinephrine and thyroxine stimulate NST. Brown adipose production begins around 26 to 28 weeks of gestation and continues until 3 to 5 weeks after delivery. Premature infants have limited amounts of brown fat and limited ability to create heat via NST.

Kangaroo Care

Dr. Edgar Ray invented **kangaroo care** in the late 1970's in Bogotá, Columbia, when morbidity and mortality rates rose in his NICU, but he had limited technological resources. Kangaroo Care consists of placing the infant, after drying and warming, in minimal clothing in an upright position on the mother's bare chest between her breasts. This allows for skin-to-skin contact with the infant's head next to the mother's heart. A precipitous drop was noted in premature infant mortality after this method of care was instigated. The concept is to provide the neonate with closeness similar to that experienced with the mother while in the womb. Kangaroo care is maintained for as long as the neonate allows. Preterm infants attached to ventilators and IV infusions also benefit from kangaroo care. There are physiological and psychological benefits for both the neonate and the mother.

Enhanced bonding between the neonate and the mother, shorter hospital stays, low cost, and decreased morbidity and mortality are all documented benefits.

Neonate's Benefits	Mother's Benefits	Institutional Benefits
Regulation of temperature, heart and respiratory rates. Calming effect with decreased stress. Decreased episodes of apnea. Increased weight gain. Enhanced bonding with the mother. Fewer nosocomial infections.	Enhanced bonding with the infant. Increased production of breast milk with higher rates of successful breast feeding. Increased confidence in caring for the infant. Increased opportunity for teaching and assessing maternal care by nursing staff.	Earlier discharge from hospital. Decreased morbidity and mortality (especially in developing countries). Decreased use of financial resources.

Skin Temperature Probes

Skin temperature probes are often used to monitor the temperature of the infant in an Isolette or radiant warmer. Incorrect placement of the probe can alter the reading, causing the warming device to deliver too much or too little heat. The temperature probe should not be placed over a bony area of the body or over an area where brown adipose tissue is abundant. Brown adipose tissue is abundant around the neck, the midscapular region of the back, the mediastinum and organs in the thoracic cavity, kidneys, and adrenal glands. A common probe placement area for an infant who is supine is over the liver. If the probe is not making good skin contact, it will indicate that the infant is cold, and the warmer will deliver increased amounts of heat, possibly causing hyperthermia. If the probe is underneath the infant, it may indicate an artificially warm temperature and decrease heat to the infant, causing hypothermia.

Neutral Thermal Environment

A **neutral thermal environment** (NTE) is a place in which the infant's body temperature is maintained within a normal range without alterations in metabolic rate or increased oxygen consumption (i.e., environmental temperature in which oxygen consumption and glucose consumption are lowest). Infants who are in an NTE are not utilizing energy to maintain their body temperature in the normal range. Just because an infant has a normal body temperature does not mean he/she is in an NTE. The infant may still be utilizing mechanisms, such as non-shivering thermogenesis, to maintain body temperatures, as evidenced by increased oxygen consumption and poor weight gain over time. Charts are commercially available that outline the appropriate NTE for infants based on current weight and birth weight.

Cold Stress/Hypothermia

Cold stress/hypothermia in the neonate is a body temperature measurement of less than 36.5° C rectally with associated symptoms. Preterm neonates are especially vulnerable to cold stress, as they have limited ability to intrinsically create or conserve body heat. They do not shiver, have limited ability to constrict superficial blood vessels and have limited amounts of both subcutaneous and brown fat. Signs of cold stress include:

- Body is cool to touch.
- Central cyanosis and acrocyanosis.
- Mottling of skin.
- Poor feeding, weak suck, increased gastric residuals, and abdominal distension.
- Bradycardia.
- Shallow respirations with tachypnea.
- Restlessness and irritability.
- Apnea.
- Lethargy and decreased activity.
- Weak cry.
- Hypoglycemia.
- Central nervous system depression with hypotonia.
- Edema.

There are a number of steps to **treatment of hypothermia**:

- Determine if the cause of hypothermia is from an abnormal physiological process in the infant or from environmental conditions.
- Do not rewarm the infant too rapidly because rapid rewarming may result in apnea or hypotension. Maintain the ambient temperature at 1 to 1.5°C higher than the infant's temperature. Oxygen consumption is not elevated when the difference between the skin temperatures and the environmental air temperature is less than 1.5°C.
- Increase the air temperature by approximately 1°C every hour until the infant's temperature is in the normal range and stable.
- Warm IV fluids with a blood-warming device prior to infusion to enhance warming.
- Closely monitor the infant's blood glucose levels, vital signs, and urinary output during rewarming.

Hyperthermia

Hyperthermia (rectal temperature greater than 37.0 °C) can be caused by excessive heat from an external source (such as a radiant warmer set too high) or internally from a hypermetabolic state (such as a fever):

External heat source	Hypermetabolic
Core temperature < skin temperature. Skin warm and flushed.	Core temperature > skin temperature. Skin cool to touch.

Infants who are physiologically competent attempt to cool themselves when hyperthermia is caused by an external heat source by an extended posture, diaphoresis, and flushed, warm skin. Hyperthermia in the neonate can cause increased metabolic demands, vasodilatation, and increased fluid loss. An increased metabolic demand leads to an increased oxygen requirement, hypoxia, cyanosis, and breathing irregularities, such as tachypnea. Increased glucose consumption leads to hypoglycemia and its associated signs (jitteriness, lethargy, vomiting, or seizures). Peripheral vasodilatation helps cool the infant but may cause tachycardia and hypotension. Increased fluid losses contribute to tachycardia and hypotension. Signs of shock may develop with lethargy and decreased urine output. Dehydration may also cause electrolyte abnormalities.

Resuscitation and Stabilization

Delivery Room Preparation

The nurse in the **delivery room** who is in charge of the care of the newborn needs to make sure that the room is properly prepared and equipped to handle any resuscitation needed. This preparation needs to be completed well before the birth. The nurse should make sure the radiant heater is on and heated, check the suction and oxygen connections to make sure they are working and hooked up. The nurse should make sure the bag and mask combination are working and are the correct size for the size infant expected. The nurse needs to check the laryngoscope to ensure the light is working and the blade is the correct size. She or he should also make certain that an assortment of endotracheal tubes in any possible size needed are ready and at the bedside. The nurse needs to gather all needed supplies and have everything ready at the bedside with personal protective equipment already on and ready to go.

APGAR Delivery Room Assessment

Dr. Virginia Apgar developed the **APGAR** test in 1952. APGAR stands for **A**ppearance, **P**ulse, **G**rimace, **A**ctivity, and **R**espiration. The APGAR is the first test given to a newborn. It is used as a quick evaluation of a newborn's physical condition to determine if any emergency medical care is needed and is administered 1 minute and 5 minutes after birth. The test is administered more than once, as the baby's condition may change rapidly. It may be administered for a third time 10 minutes after birth if needed. The baby is rated on the five subscales and scores added together. A total score of ≥7 is a sign of good health.

Sign	0	1	2
Appearance (Skin Color)	Cyanotic or pallor over entire body	Normal, except for the extremities	Entire body normal
Pulse (Heart Rate)	Absent	<100 bpm	>100 bpm
Grimace (Reflex Irritability)	Unresponsive	Grimace	Infant sneezes, coughs, and recoils
Activity (Muscle Tone)	Absent	Flexed limbs	Infant moves freely
Respiration (Breathing Rate and Effort)	Absent	Bradypnea, dyspnea	Good breathing and crying

Rapid Assessment

The infant should be given a **rapid assessment** within seconds of birth to determine if the infant is at term, if the amniotic fluid is clear, if there is muscle tone, and if there are respirations or crying. If any of these conditions are not met, then the child should be placed under radiant heat and further resuscitation done. The basic steps to resuscitation include:

- Warming the infant after drying.
- Positioning the infant and clearing the airway if necessary.
- Stimulating and repositioning the infant.

The child should be evaluated throughout the initial procedures:

- Respirations: Rate and character of respirations should be noted as well as observation of chest wall movement.
- Heart rate: Should be >100 bpm, assessed with stethoscope or at the base of the umbilical cord.

Minimum Neonatal Resuscitation Equipment

Temperature	Thermometer, warmed drying towels, warmed swaddling blankets, radiant warmer, phototherapy equipment
Respiration	Oxygen tank and hood, flow meter, humidifier, heater, tubing, nasal prongs Bag and mask set-up (assorted sizes) Laryngoscope with size 0 and 1 blades Endotracheal tubes, sizes 2.5-4 Bulb syringe, suction catheters, sizes 6, 8, and 10 French, suction canister Cardiorespiratory monitor, oxygen analyzer
Fluids	IV needles and tubing, infusion pump, umbilical catheters (sizes 2.5 and 5 Fr) Blood pressure monitor, pulse oximeter Isotonic saline, D10W, sodium bicarbonate If transfusions are done here, blood drainage system, volume expander, and blood warmer
Drugs	Epinephrine, Naloxone
Procedures	Various sterile surgical packs, dressings, chest tubes, scalpels, hemostat, arterial blood gas equipment and portable x-ray machine

ABCs of Infant Resuscitation

The **ABC's of resuscitation** are a device to help remember what order to do which steps of the resuscitation process. In this device, the letters stand for as follows:

- **A—Airway:** An airway should be established as the very first thing tended to, if there is no airway, air cannot be moved during resuscitation attempts. This step includes clearing the mouth and nose of secretions, and properly positioning the infant in the "sniff" position
- **B—Breathing**: This step involves initiating breathing after the airway has been established, this can be done with stimulation, supplemental oxygen or through artificial ventilation
- **C—Circulation:** Once an airway and breathing have been established, then the circulation is considered, chest compressions may be indicated here or the administration of volume expanders and possibly epinephrine.

Establishing Airway and Stimulating Respirations

To **establish an airway,** the infant is placed supine with the head slightly extended in the "sniffing" position. A small neck roll may be placed under the shoulders to maintain this position in a very small premature infant. Once the proper position is established, the mouth and nose is suctioned (mouth first to prevent reflex inspiration of secretions when nose suctioned) with a bulb syringe or catheter if necessary. The infant's head can be turned momentarily to the side to allow secretions to pool in the cheek where they can be more easily suctioned and removed to establish the airway. **Stimulating** the newborn is often all that is needed to initiate spontaneous respirations in the neonate. This tactile stimulation can be accomplished by gently rubbing the back or trunk of the infant. Another technique used to provide stimulation is flicking or rubbing the soles of the feet. Slapping neonates as stimulation is no longer practiced and should NOT be used.

Administration of Free-Flow Oxygen

If an infant remains cyanotic in the chest area (central cyanosis) after the initial steps of resuscitation have taken place, administering **free-flow oxygen** is the next step to take. Free flow oxygen is administered to the neonate by the use of either a mask hooked up to an oxygen source or by the use of the oxygen tubing itself. If the tubing alone is used, the nurse can hold the tube with a cupped hand helping to direct and concentrate the oxygen at the infant's airway. Free flow oxygen should be administered at a rate of 5 L/minute. If the infant starts to turn pink, the oxygen can be carefully and slowly removed while continuing to closely monitor the infant for returning cyanosis. If the infant remains centrally cyanotic after the administration of free-flow oxygen, bag and mask ventilation must be considered as the next step.

Bag and Mask Ventilation

Ventilation using a **bag and mask** is indicated when one or more of the following occurs and has not responded to other resuscitation attempts:

- Apnea that does not respond to tactile stimulation such as rubbing the chest or back or flicking the soles of the feet.
- Gasping respirations.
- Heart rate of less than 100 beats per minute, determined by auscultation at the apex of the heart or palpation of the base of the umbilical cord.
- Central cyanosis that persists after administering free-flow oxygen, acrocyanosis alone is NOT an indication for the need for further oxygenation or ventilation.

The flowmeter is set at 5-10 L/minute, and opening breath pressures of 30-40 cm H_2O are used for term infants and 20-25 cm H_2O for preterm. Ventilation is done at 40-60 breaths/minute with pressure of 15-20 cm H_2O for normal lungs and 20-50 cm H_2O for immature or compromised lungs.

Gastric Suctioning

When an infant has been resuscitated using a bag and mask, air is inadvertently pumped into the stomach as it is being pumped into the lungs, so **gastric suctioning** is necessary. Once respirations have been stabilized either spontaneously or with mechanical ventilation, the stomach should be aspirated to remove any air pumped into it. If the air is left in the abdomen, it causes there to be an upward pressure on the lungs from the distended abdomen, this compromises lung capacity and breathing effort. An orogastric catheter or size 8 Fr. feeding tube is inserted by measuring the distance from the nose to the earlobe then to the xiphoid, marking the tube at this distance then advancing it to the mark. A 20 mL syringe is then attached to the tube and the contents of the stomach aspirated. Once all the air or fluid is aspirated, the tube is left in place open to air and taped to the infant's cheek. This will keep the stomach decompressed of air.

Chest Compressions

If **chest compressions** are indicated for resuscitation, the following steps should be followed:

- Position the neonate in the "sniffing" position with the neck slightly extended.
- Make sure there is firm support for the infant's back.

- Using a two-finger technique proceed with the compressions on the lower third of the sternum at a rate of **90 times per minute a**nd with a depth of one third of the anterior posterior diameter of the chest.
- When performing the compressions, the hands should be placed in a circle around the chest to provide support to the infants back.
- The ratio of compressions to breaths should be 3 to 1.
- Check the heart rate again after 30 seconds of compressions (about 45 compressions total).
- If heart rate is less than 60 beats per minute, continue with another round of compressions but if the rate is 60 beats per minute or higher then compressions can stop.

Providing Warmth

Infants have poor temperature regulation ability, particularly preterm infants who lack brown fat, which is one of the body's tools to regulate body temperature, so **providing warmth** is critical as a component of resuscitation. An infant who is just seconds old and wet will need aggressive measures to keep it warm while any resuscitation efforts are being initiated. Infants lose heat through their head so one of the first steps should be to place a hat on the head. The infant should be placed under a radiant heater and vigorous drying with warmed blankets should begin. Often this stimulation, drying and warming is all that is needed to establish a regular respiration pattern in the neonate. Preterm infants weighing <1500 grams should be placed in a plastic bag (made specifically for this purpose) up to the height of the shoulders to prevent cold shock. A term infant with no apparent distress can be placed on the mother's chest and covered with a warm blanket.

Stress Related to Light

Light is a necessary component of caring for both the sick and healthy neonate in the delivery room and nursery. Adequate lighting is required to evaluate the at-risk neonate, to assess color, to complete procedures such as intubation, or to give medications. Light discourages the growth of pathogens. However, constant bright light interferes with the development of natural diurnal rhythms because it arouses the central nervous system and stresses the infant. Controlling light helps to stabilize the infant. Some simple methods to protect the neonate from light over-stimulation and to establish a normal sleep cycle include:

- Reducing overhead light levels when direct visualization is not necessary.
- Covering incubator hoods to reduce light entering the incubator.
- Dimming the lights at night to help establish a natural day/night pattern (circadian rhythm).

Sress Related to Noise

Excessive **noise** causes agitation in both term and especially preterm neonates. The preterm neonate has less ability to self-calm, and over-stimulation results in decompensation, as demonstrated by increased oxygen requirements and increased apnea and bradycardia episodes. The American Academy of Pediatrics (AAP) recommends noise levels in the nursery and NICU be kept at ≥45 decibels. A normal speaking voice is between 50 to 60 decibels. Noise levels above 80 to 85 decibels damage the cochlea and cause hearing loss in adults. To keep noise acceptably low:

- Turn radios/TVs off or down.
- Designate a daily quiet time.
- Close incubator portholes gently, because closing a plastic porthole can spike the decibel level more than 80 dB.

- *Whisper* — avoid speaking loudly.
- Remove bubbling water from ventilator tubing.
- Educate parents about the deleterious effects of over-stimulating their infant with loud noises.

Environmental Stressors and "Time Out"

Premature neonates have a very limited ability to deal with **environmental stressors,** but these stressors can affect all neonates. Signs of stress in neonates include:

- Color changes, such as mottling or cyanosis.
- Episodes of apnea and bradycardia.
- Activity changes, such as tremors, twitches, frantic activity, arching, and gaze averting.
- Flaccid posture (sagging trunk, extremities and face).
- Easy fatigability.

When the infant shows signs of stress, a **"time out"** recovery period is indicated:

- Stop the activity causing the stress.
- Reduce unnecessary stimuli, e.g., lower the lights and postpone non-essential manipulation of the neonate.
- Give the neonate a chance to calm or soothe himself.
- Bundle the neonate and place him/her in a comforting, side-lying position with the shoulders drawn forward and the hands brought to midline.

Non-Nutritive Sucking

Nonnutritive sucking occurs when an infant sucks on an item such as a pacifier, or his/her own fist. Nonnutritive sucking is not associated with nutritional intake, but it is an important method of self-quieting and begins in the uterus at about 29 weeks of gestation. Extremely premature infants often lack basic neurodevelopmental capabilities, and cannot coordinate sucking, swallowing, and breathing simultaneously. Typically, the ability to suck and swallow in a coordinated fashion is not present until 32 to 34 weeks of gestation. Premature infants should be encouraged to perform non-nutritive sucking during the gavage feeding process if they can accomplish it. Benefits of nonnutritive sucking include:

- Improved digestion of enteral feeds because digestive enzyme release is stimulated.
- Facilitated development of coordinated nutritive sucking behavior.
- Calming of the distressed infant.

Proper Positioning of the Premature Neonate

Correct positioning of the premature neonate minimizes outside stimuli and mimics the enclosed and calming environment of the womb, helping with the transition to extrauterine life:

- Place the neonate in a flexed position, with his hands close to midline and near his face.
- Create a nest of blankets or pillows to:
  o Help block out light and noise.
  o Give him the impression of a closed environment.
  o Minimize abnormal molding of the head from prolonged pressure on one side.
- Cover the incubator to further keep out sound and light.

- Place the neonate in the prone position (on his stomach) to help to stabilize the chest wall, improves ventilation, and increases the amount of time an infant is in quiet sleep. However, infants should be placed supine (on the back) most of the time, to decrease the chance of SIDS.

Cord Blood Gas Interpretation

Umbilical cord blood gas testing, preferably arterial, should be done ≥60 minutes of birth for infants who are at risk or depressed to determine pH and acid-base balance. Testing is most applicable to infants with low APGAR scores (0-3) persisting for ≥5 minutes. A pH of <7 may indicate birth asphyxia/hypoxia severe enough to cause neurological deficits. Infants with normal APGAR scores may also have pH <7 but without pathology, so results must be evaluated in relation to the APGAR scores and child's general condition. Preterm infants often have low APGAR scores and may be suspected of having birth asphyxia, but if they have suffered no birth asphyxia or hypoxia, the pH level usually remains normal.

Normal cord blood values			Abnormal cord blood values	
	Venous	**Arterial**	**Respiratory Acidosis**	**Metabolic acidosis**
pH	7.25 to 7.35	7.28	<7.25	<7.25
pO$_2$	28-32 mm Hg.	16-20 mm Hg.	Varies	<20 mm Hg.
PCO$_2$	40-50 mm Hg.	40-50 mm Hg.	>50 mm Hg.	44 to 55 mm Hg.
Base excess	0 to 5 mEq/L	0-10 mEq/L	< 10 mEq/L	>10mEq/L

Birth Asphyxia

Birth asphyxia is the cause of many problems after birth. Birth asphyxia is defined as an event that alters the exchange of gas (oxygen and carbon dioxide). This interference with gas exchange leads to a decrease in the amount of oxygen delivered to the fetus along with an increase in the level of carbon dioxide the fetus is exposed to. This gas imbalance causes the fetus to switch from normal aerobic metabolism to anaerobic metabolism. Fetal distress results and this distress then leads to increased fetal heart rate, release of meconium into the amniotic fluid, and lowered pH. Infants experiencing birth asphyxia will often present at birth with APGAR scores that are less than 5. Symptoms of birth asphyxia include:

- *Mild:* Overly alert for the first 45 minutes to one hour following birth (infants are normally sleepy after about 15 minutes following birth). The pupils are dilated. The respiratory rate and the heart rate will both be slightly increased. Newborn reflexes and muscle tone are normal. Oxygen may be administered.
- Moderate:
  - Hypothermia as evidenced by low body temperature.
  - Hypoglycemia as glucose store are used up trying to supply organs needed energy.
  - Pupils are constricted.
  - Signs of respiratory distress are evident.
  - May experience seizure activity at 12-24 hours of age.
  - Lethargy (floppy infant).
  - Bradycardia
- **Severe**: This requires close monitoring in a NICU and symptoms would include:
  - Pale color related to the inability of the heart to perfuse the body.
  - Cerebral edema related to apnea episodes and/or intracranial hemorrhage.

Resuscitation will vary according to the infant's condition, but warming the infant, stabilizing the glucose level, and providing oxygen or EMCO (in severe cases) may be indicated.

Meconium in Amniotic Fluid

When **meconium is present in the amniotic fluid**, the following steps should be taken immediately following birth to avoid meconium aspiration syndrome:

- If the infant is crying and showing no signs of distress, the mouth, nose and throat should be suctioned with a suction catheter and the usual steps of drying and stimulation completed.
- If the infant shows signs of respiratory distress in the presence of meconium stained fluid, the infant should be immediately intubated with an endotracheal tube for the purpose of suctioning the trachea. Once intubated, the trachea can be suctioned with a large catheter attached to wall suction.
- Once the airway has been adequately suctioned and cleared, the stomach may need to be suctioned as well in order to prevent the regurgitation of the swallowed meconium. Meconium that is swallowed and then regurgitated can be aspirated into the lungs.

Naloxone Hydrochloride

Naloxone hydrochloride, an opiate antagonist, is not used in the routine resuscitation of an infant but is used in one very specific situation following birth. Naloxone is considered the antidote for narcotics administered to the mother of the infant within 4 hours of birth if the infant shows signs of serious respiratory depression from secondary absorption. If the mother of the infant has narcotics in her system as a result of an addiction to narcotics rather than as treatment for labor pain, however, Naloxone cannot be given to this infant. If Naloxone is given to an infant born to a narcotic addicted mother, the drug will cause a severe abstinence reaction in the newborn that can result in seizure.

Neonatal Transport

An infant that is severely compromised at birth or <32 weeks gestation often require **transport** to specialized neonatal care units, usually because of respiratory distress, preterm birth, congenital anomalies, and suspected cardiac abnormalities. The infant should be resuscitated and stabilized prior to transport. Communication with the regional center should be immediate and detailed. The **STABLE program** (sugar, temperature, artificial breathing, blood pressure, lab work, and emotional support) can guide efforts to stabilize the infant. The transport team must take copies of all records and lab reports. Transport teams may include NICU nurses, NNPs, physicians, and respiratory therapists. Adequate supplies (similar to those needed for resuscitation) must be available as well as oxygen, air-blended mixtures, monitors and transport incubators. The incubator must control temperature while allowing access. Insulating material may be needed for very cold environments.

Nutrition

Digestion and Absorption

Digestion comprises the processes by which food is converted into chemicals that are used by the body. These processes are immature at birth and most don't function until 3-6 months. Digestion begins in the mouth as milk is mixed with saliva, but salivary amylase, which begins digestion of starch, has little effect on milk because it passes into the esophagus and stomach quickly. Protein digestion begins in the stomach where hydrochloric acid acts on curds formed by the enzyme renin.

The curds slow the progress of the milk to allow digestion. Pancreatic and liver enzymes further digest protein and fat in the small intestine. Infants cannot adequately absorb fat until 4-5 months or complex carbohydrates until 4-6 months. Simple carbohydrates break down into glucose and monosaccharides and fat into fatty acids and glycerol. Trypsin levels are sufficient to convert proteins into polypeptides and amino acids. **Absorption**, the transfer of digestive end products (electrolytes, vitamins, fluids, nutrients) into the circulation, takes place primarily in the small intestine and is facilitated by villi.

Caloric Requirements

The **caloric needs** of a neonate (pre-term or term) depend on postnatal age, activity, current weight, growth rate, thermal environment, and route of nutritional intake. Cold stress increases caloric requirements. Infants who receive parenteral nutrition need fewer calories as they do not have any fecal loss, and the nutrients are not absorbed by the gastrointestinal tract. The general requirements for adequate growth include:

- Full term infant: 100 to 120 cal/kg/day.
- Premature infants: 110 to 160 cal/kg/day.
- Infants who are recovering from surgery or have a chronic illness, such as bronchopulmonary dysplasia (BPD): ≥180 cal/kg/day.

Unfortified formulas (and most breast milk) supply 20 calories per ounce. To ingest 120 cal/kg/day, an infant needs to ingest 6 ounces/kg/day of unfortified formula or breast milk. Special formulas designed for premature infants and fortifiers that can be added to breast milk provide higher calorie contents per ounce (22 to 24 calories per ounce).

Protein Requirements

Neonates require adequate **protein intake** to sustain growth. Protein requirements depend on gestational age. A positive nitrogen balance exists when the intake of protein meets or exceeds the infant's requirements. A negative protein balance occurs when protein is provided in inadequate amounts and can lead to catabolism (muscle breakdown). Premature neonates have higher protein requirements than full term infants:

- Full term: 2 to 2.5 g/kg/day.
- Preterm: 3.5 to 4 g/kg/day.

Preterm infants should be started on parenteral nutrition supplemented with protein as soon as possible to avoid negative protein balances. Special formulas designed for premature infants are available with elevated protein contents. Breast milk fortifiers are also available to enhance the protein levels and caloric content of breast milk for premature infants although the content of breast milk adjusts automatically for the needs of preterm infants.

Carbohydrates, Fats, and Proteins

Carbohydrates: One gram of carbohydrates provides 3.4 calories. Carbohydrates should provide approximately 40-50% of total daily calories. Lactose is the predominant carbohydrate. Premature infants may be deficient in the enzyme lactase (enzyme that breaks down lactose), so premature infant formulas utilize lesser amounts of lactose, combined with glucose polymers.

Fat: One gram of fat provides 9 calories. Lipids should supply approximately 40-52% of total daily calories. Common sources of lipids include palm, soybean, coconut, and safflower oils. Premature infant formulas have a higher percentage of fat supplied as medium-chain triglycerides (MCT). MCTs can be absorbed without pancreatic lipase or bile salts that are deficient in premature infants.

Proteins: One gram of protein provides 4 calories. Proteins should provide less than 5% of total daily calories. Proteins provide amino acids that are used as building blocks for muscle and other tissues. Preterm formulas have higher protein content than term formula to help meet the increased growth requirements of preterm infants.

Enteral Feeding

Enteral (tube) feeding provides nutrition to infants with a functioning gastrointestinal tract but the inability to take an adequate amount of milk/formula orally. Ideally, human milk is provided for enteral feedings because it provides antimicrobial factors (IgA, leukocytes, complement, lactoferrin, lysozyme) lacking in formula. However, preterm infants don't grow at adequate rates on human milk alone, so human milk is usually supplemented with formula that contains additional carbohydrates, protein, fatty acids, vitamins, and minerals. Enteral feeding is indicated in infants requiring endotracheal intubation, or weak infants with inability to suck, swallow, or gag reflex or coordinate these activities (<34-36 weeks). Feedings may be continuous or intermittent (over 30 to 60 minutes). Feedings should be given slowly and tube position checked frequently to prevent aspiration. If feedings must be prolonged, oral aversion and gastroesophageal reflux may occur, so gastrostomy tube placement may be done. Oral feedings must be introduced slowly once per day, then once per 8 hours, every third feeding, every other feeding, and finally every meal.

A feeding tube for **enteral feeding** should be measured (tip of ear to midpoint between xiphoid process and umbilicus) and marked before insertion. The infant should be swaddled and supine. Oral tubes are used for infants <1 kg and those with NCPAP, ventilator, or high need for oxygen. Nasal tubes are used for infants >1kg or those taking oral feedings or with strong gag reflex. Short-term tubes (polyvinyl chloride) are changed every 24-72 hours and long-term tubes (polyurethane) every month. Prior to feeding, stomach contents are aspirated for assessment but then re-instilled to prevent electrolyte loss unless blood, bile, stool, or thick mucous is in aspirate. Feeding should be by gravity flow 5-8 inches above infant, usually over 30 minutes for intermittent feeding, and the tube should be cleared with 1-2 mL water at end. For continuous feeding, the placement of the tube and residual milk/formula should be checked every 2 hours. Usually, a 4-hour amount of milk/formula feeding is hung at one time.

Trophic Feedings

Trophic feedings (also called minimal enteric nutrition) are very small enteral feeds given soon after birth to extremely premature infants not expected to tolerate enteral feeds for several weeks. Studies have shown that trophic feeds prevent atrophy of the gut and enhance gastrointestinal maturation and small intestine motility. They may also protect the preterm infants from developing necrotizing enterocolitis (NEC). Trophic feeds can be started within 24 to 48 hours of birth in stable infants. The fluids of choice are colostrum, human breast milk, or preterm infant formula. Trophic feedings are non-nutritive (not designed to add significant calories or nutrition to the infant). Typical volumes are 1 to 2 ml/kg per feeding, with a total volume not to exceed 15 ml/kg/day.

Total Parenteral Nutrition

A preterm or compromised infant may not tolerate enteral feedings for several weeks, so the infant's nutritional needs are met with IV **total parenteral nutrition** (TPN). The goals of TPN are to:

- Provide normal metabolism.
- Support growth without significant morbidity.
- Prevent essential fatty acid deficiency.
- Balance nitrogen.
- Prevent muscle wasting (catabolism).

TPN is started after birth. Dextrose provides the majority of calories, but to avoid elevated blood glucose levels, dextrose is administered at 6mg/kg/min and increased to 10 to 12 mg/kg/min over several days. The infant's serum glucose is monitored regularly for hyperglycemia. Protein content is slowly increased over several days to 3 to 3.5 g/kg/day. Lipids, required for calories and the absorption of fat-soluble vitamins like A, D, and E, are started at 0.5/gm/kg/day and increased to 3 to 3.5 gm/kg/day. Other components of TPN include sodium, potassium, calcium, phosphorus, magnesium, trace elements, and vitamins. TPN may be administered through a peripheral IV line for <one week and a central line for longer periods.

Intravenous Lipids

Intravenous lipids are an important component of total parenteral nutrition (TPN) because they provide essential fatty acids, a concentrated calorie source (9 calories per gram of fat), and improve delivery of fat-soluble vitamins to infants who cannot tolerate enteral feeds. General guidelines for the administration of IV lipids are to start with 0.5/g/kg on the third day of life and advance slowly to a final administration rate of 3 to 3.5/g/kg/day by 7 to 10 days. Delivery of IV lipids should be continuous over 18 to 24 hours each day. Serum lipid levels should be monitored for hyperlipidemia. Potential complications include:

- Risk of kernicterus in infants with elevated unconjugated bilirubin. Free fatty acids displace bilirubin from albumin binding sites. Infusion of lipids should be at the lower level in infants with elevated unconjugated bilirubin.
- Exacerbation of chronic lung disease.
- Exacerbation of persistent pulmonary hypertension.

Complications Associated with TPN

Complications of total parenteral nutrition (TPN) result from the presence of the intravenous access (usually a central line) and the development of cholestasis. Both of these events are more common in infants receiving TPN longer than 2 to 3 weeks. The longer an infant receives TPN, the more likely complications will occur. Consequences of prolonged venous access include sepsis, thrombophlebitis, and extravasation of fluid into soft tissue with possible tissue necrosis. Premature infants have an immature hepatobiliary system. One hypothesis for the development of cholestasis is that a lack of fat in the duodenum leads to biliary stasis. Infants requiring TPN are often very ill, may have episodes of shock, or require surgical interventions, all of which contribute to the development of TPN-associated cholestasis. Jaundiced infants show an elevated direct bilirubin in blood serum. Treatment usually involves the discontinuation of TPN, along with the slow introduction of enteral feeds (if possible).

Breast Milk

Breast milk is the food of choice for newborn infants:

- It provides the appropriate amounts of carbohydrate, protein, fat, vitamins, minerals, enzymes, and trace elements.
- It contains antibodies from the mother that help bolster the infant's immature immune system.
- Breast fed babies have reduced risks of eczema, asthma, obesity, and elevated cholesterol later in life.
- Breastfeeding enhances the bond between the mother and the infant by physical contact and learning to recognize communication signals.
- The maternal cost is an extra 500 calories a day and extra water.
- There is no chance of causing kidney damage by mixing formula incorrectly.

Colostrum, produced during the first few days after birth, is scant, thick, yellowish, and high in protein and antibody content. Colostrum stimulates the passage of meconium. Transitional milk is thinner and white with a composition closer to mature milk. By the third or fourth day after birth, the mother produces 23-27 ounces of bluish-white, mature breast milk.

Breast milk has immunologic benefits that formulas lack, resulting in decreased morbidity in breast-fed infants. Breast milk contains:

- *Antibodies*: Secretory IgA to provide protection from respiratory, enteric, and viral pathogens.
- *Primary nutrients:* Protein with whey to casein ratio of 60:40 (including IgM, IgG, lactoferrin, lysozyme, casein [40%], and fibronectin), carbohydrate (about 40% of total calories), and fat (free fatty acids).

Secondary nutrients:

- Nucleotides.
- Vitamins A, C, D, E. Vitamin D content is $\geq$25 IU/L so infants need supplementation $\geq$2 months of age.
- Enzymes: Antiinflammatory and antibacterial properties. Includes lipase, which breaks down fat.
- Growth factors.
- Hormones: Prolactin, cortisol, thyroxine, insulin and erythropoietin.
- Cells: β-lymphocytes, macrophages (90%), neutrophil, T-lymphocytes, cytokines, interleukin 1b, 6, 8, 10, 12 (providing both inflammatory and anti-inflammatory properties).

Special Preterm Formulas

Preterm formulas are designed with the special requirements of the premature infant in mind. These infants often have an increased caloric requirement to meet growth expectations. Preterm formulas differ from full term formulas because they provide:

- 24 cal/ounce as opposed to the 20 cal/ounce found in breast milk and formulas for full term infants.
- Increased levels of protein, vitamins, and minerals, particularly increased amounts of vitamin D, calcium, and phosphorus to prevent osteopenia of prematurity.
- Less lactose than term formulas, so they are less likely to cause diarrhea.

Breast milk can be "fortified" with the addition of human milk fortifiers (HMF) to achieve the same results. Infants are typically switched to a transitional or cow milk-based formula prior to discharge.

Fat-Soluble Vitamins in Formulas

Vitamins found in formulas are organic nutrients required in small amounts to maintain growth and normal metabolism. **Fat-soluble vitamins** include:

- ***Vitamin A:*** Important for growth and development of tissues and in proper functioning of the immune system. Vitamin A supplementation in extremely low birth weight infants has been shown to reduce the incidence of bronchopulmonary dysplasia.
- ***Vitamin D***: Required for adequate calcium and phosphorus absorption. Vitamin D deficiency leads to rickets (soft bones, bowed legs).
- ***Vitamin E:*** An antioxidant that is limited in preterm infants, making them susceptible to developing hemolytic anemia without proper supplementation.
- ***Vitamin K***: Important in the clotting process. Infants receive an injection of Vitamin K shortly after birth to prevent hemorrhagic disease of the newborn.

Excessive fat-soluble vitamins A and D are toxic because they accumulate in adipose tissue and the liver. Water-soluble vitamins include thiamine (B_1), riboflavin (B_2), niacin (B_3), pantothenate (B_5), pyridoxine (B_6), cobalamin (B_{12}), C, biotin, and folic acid. Excessive water-soluble vitamins are excreted in the urine.

Soy vs. Dairy Formulas

Energy Source	Soy Formulas	Cow's Milk Formulas
Carbohydrate	Sucrose	Lactose
Protein	Soy isolate from the soy bean	Whey and casein in various ratios (similar to breast milk)

Pros of Soy Use	Cons of Soy Use
Soy is appropriate for use in infants with: Hereditary galactosemia and hereditary lactase deficiency. Documented IgE mediated allergy to cow's milk protein. Temporary lactase deficiency that may occur after infectious gastroenteritis. Parents who are seeking a vegetarian-based diet.	Soy cannot be used for premature infants weighing less than 1,800 grams because it results in: Less weight gain. Less linear growth. Increased risk for developing osteopenia. Elevated levels of alkaline phosphatase. Elevated levels of aluminum. Phytoestrogens found in soy formulas may alter normal endocrine patterns of the infant.

Pregestimil®, Similac® PM 60/40, and Nutramigen® LIPL

Pregestimil® is a hypoallergenic formula specially designed for infants with malabsorption caused by gastrointestinal or hepatobiliary disease. It provides hydrolyzed (predigested) protein that is easier to digest. The majority of the fats are in the form of medium chain triglycerides (MCT). MCTs are easier to digest than other forms of fats.

Similac® PM 60/40 is a cow's milk-based formula that has a low phosphorus content and low renal solute load. It is designed for infants with impaired renal function or with hypocalcemia due to hyperphosphatemia. It has a whey-to-casein ratio of 60:40.

Nutramigen® LIPL is a hypoallergenic formula designed for infants sensitive to the intact protein found in cow's milk-based formula. The proteins are hydrolyzed (digested) and easier to absorb. Cow's milk protein allergy is an indication for use of this formula. It contains docosahexaenoic (DHA) acid and arachidonic acid (ARA) that are also found in breast milk. DHA and ARA are omega 3 and 6 fatty acids that support normal brain, eye, and nerve development.

Carnitine Supplementation

Carnitine is a quaternary amino acid that is synthesized from methionine and lysine in the liver and kidney. Carnitine aids in the metabolism of long chain fatty acids by helping to transport them across the mitochondrial membrane. Carnitine is present in human breast milk and formulas in sufficient amounts. Infants who are premature have low tissue stores of carnitine, as much of it is transferred to the fetus during the third trimester. Symptoms of carnitine deficiency include increased episodes of apnea, decreased muscle tone, and poor growth. Infants who are not being enterally fed and are receiving TPN may benefit from supplementation with carnitine because it makes them better able to metabolize fats.

Iron Supplementation

The premature infant is especially susceptible to iron deficiency because of the lack of maternal iron transfer during the third trimester and the multiple blood samplings that occur with the extensive monitoring of the premature infant. To minimize the risk of iron deficiency anemia, premature infants fed human milk should be started on **iron supplementation** once they receive full enteral feeds. Studies have shown that premature infants fed a premature formula have better iron stores when that formula is supplemented with 15 mg/L of iron vs. those receiving formula with 3 mg/L of iron. All formula-fed term infants should receive iron-fortified formulas. Breastfed term infants should be given iron supplementation when they are several months old.

Fluids and Electrolytes

Renal System and Fluid Maintenance

Maintenance of adequate fluid volume can be difficult in neonates. The pediatric renal system matures over the first 3 years of life. The nephrons in the young infant's kidneys are immature and the glomerular filtration rate is low because of impaired ability to filter urine until about 6-12 months of age. Also, the ability to concentrate or dilute urine may not reach adult levels until ages 2-3 years. Premature infants may have additional renal abnormalities, such as decreased creatinine clearance or impaired sodium retention. Infants are less tolerant of both dehydration and fluid overload. The 4-2-1 rule is used to determine maintenance fluid requirements:

- 4 mL/kg/hr for first 10 kg weight, 2 mL/kg/hr for second 10 kg, and 1 mL/kg/hr for remaining kgs.

Often a programmable infusion pump or buret with microdrip is used to manage fluids because the balance must be maintained within a narrow range.

Body Fluid/Fluid Balance

Body fluid is primarily intracellular fluid (ICF) or extracellular space (ECF). Infants and children have proportionately more extracellular fluid (ECF) than adults. At birth, more than half of the child's weight is ECF (by 3 years of age, the balance is more like adults):

- ECF: 20-30% (intrastitial fluid, plasma, transcellular fluid).
- ICF: 40-50% (fluid within the cells).

The fluid compartments are separated by semipermeable membranes that allow fluid and solutes (electrolytes and other substances) to move by osmosis. Fluid also moves through diffusion, filtration, and active transport. In fluid volume deficit, fluid is out of balance and ECF is depleted; an overload occurs with increased concentration of sodium and retention of fluid. Signs of fluid deficit include:

- Restless to lethargic.
- Increasing pulse rate, tachycardia.
- Fontanels depressed.
- ↓ Urinary output.
- Normal BP progressing hypotension.
- Dry mucous membranes, thirst.
- ↓ in body weight.

Total Body Water

Total body water (TBW) content is the percentage of the body composed of water. An extremely premature infant (24 to 26 weeks of gestation) has a TBW content of 90%. The TBW content drops to 75-80% at full term (40 weeks), compared to 60-65% in adults. Because preterm infants have such a high percentage of TBW, any fluid loss can cause severe problems. Physiological diuresis is fluid loss from the extracellular space, and this is the initial type of fluid loss in neonates. Because intracellular space is relatively small in neonates, there is less fluid available to shift into the extracellular space, so the effects of extracellular fluid loss are much more pronounced on infants than adults. Diuresis continues during the first week after birth, so full term infants lose 5-10% of their weight, and premature infants lose 10-15% of their weight. Diuresis diminishes but slowly continues over the first 1 to 2 years of life. The typical toddler has a TBW content of 60%.

Preterm Neonatal Urinary Output

The pre-term neonate has 3 phases of **urine output**:

1. ***Oliguric phase:*** Output is lower than intake during the first 12 to 24 hours after birth. The premature infant's urine output may be less than 1 ml/kg/hr in the oliguric phase.
2. ***Diuretic phase:*** Output is greater than intake 24 to 72 hours after birth. The premature infant's urine output may be greater than 5 ml/kg/hr in the diuretic phase, so the infant's weight decreases.
3. ***Adaptive phase:*** Output is appropriate after 72 hours, as the kidneys adjust to the rate of input. The urine output more closely reflects the real fluid status of the infant.

The appropriate response to decreased fluid intake is to decrease urine output and produce concentrated urine (elevate the specific gravity). The appropriate response to excessive fluids is to increase urine output and produce dilute urine (lower the specific gravity).

Fluid Deficit

Pediatric fluid deficit must also be carefully estimated and managed. Fluid deficit should be replaced over 3 hours with half the first hour and a quarter in the remaining 2 hours. Fluid deficit is calculated by first finding the ***maintenance fluid requirement***:

- Maintenance fluid mL X hours NPO = fluid deficit.

Preoperative deficits usually are treated with lactated Ringer's or 1/ normal saline (which may cause hyperchloremic acidosis). Glucose containing fluids may contribute to hyperglycemia.

Fluid replacement must account for both blood loss and third-space loss:

- Blood: Replacement may be with lactated Ringers (3 mL to 1 mL blood loss) or 5% albumin colloid (1 mL to 1 mL blood loss) to maintain hematocrit at predetermined adequate minimal level:
  o Infants and neonates: >30% (may be as high as 40-50%).
  o Older children: 20-26%.

Blood is replaced with packed red blood cells when the allowable blood loss threshold is exceeded.

Allowable blood loss is calculated by the following formula based on the infant's average hematocrit:

- Average hematocrit = (Beginning hematocrit + minimum adequate hematocrit) / 2.
- Allowable blood loss = [Estimated blood loss X (beginning hematocrit − minimum adequate hematocrit)] / average hematocrit.

Blood loss should be monitored carefully to determine when it exceeds the allowable blood loss. ***Volume of packed red blood cell replacement*** is based on the hematocrit of packed cells, 75%:

- Packed red blood cells in mL = [Estimated blood loss − allowable blood loss) X minimum adequate hematocrit] / packed red blood cell hematocrit of 75.

If blood loss is in excess of 1-2 blood volumes, then 10-15 mL/kg of platelets and FFP are administered. **Third space loss** after surgery can only be estimated based on the degree of trauma:

- Minor: 3-4 mL/kg/hr; Moderate: 5-6 mL/kg/hr; Severe: 7-10 mL/kg/hr.

Lactated Ringers is most commonly used to replace third space loss.

Sodium, Hyponatremia, and Hypernatremia

Sodium (Na) regulates fluid volume, osmolality, acid-base balance, and activity in the muscles, nerves and myocardium. It is the primary cation (positive ion) in ECF, necessary to maintain ECF levels needed for tissue perfusion:

- Normal neonatal value: 133-146 mEq/L.
- Hyponatremia: <133 mEq/L. (Critical value <120).
- Hypernatremia: >146 mEq/L. (Critical value >160).

Hyponatremia develops with excessive water gain or excessive sodium loss. Late symptoms include apnea, irritability, twitching, and seizures when serum sodium drops below 120 mEq/L, but infants are often asymptomatic. In the first days after birth, hyponatremia is usually secondary to excessive water gain (dilutional hyponatremia), reflected in a weight gain or absence of expected weight loss. Conditions causing dilutional hyponatremia include syndrome of inappropriate antidiuretic hormone (SIADH), renal dysfunction with decreased urine output, and overhydration. Treatment involves identifying and treating underlying cause, restricting fluid, and replacing sodium if necessary. ***Hypernatremia*** is caused by dehydration, excess use of sodium containing solutions, and diabetes insipidus. Late symptoms include seizures. Underlying cause must be identified and treated.

Calcium and Hypocalcemia

The ionized form of serum **calcium** is the only biologically available form in the body:

- Cord: 8.2-11.2 mg/dL.
- 0-10 days: 7.6-10.4 mg/dL.
- 11 days to 1 yrs: 9.0-11.0 mg/dL.
- Critical value for hypocalcemia: <7 mg/dL

Signs of ***hypocalcemia*** include jitteriness, irritability, stridor, tetany, high-pitched cry, seizures, and decreased myocardial contractility with decreased cardiac output. An electrocardiogram may show a prolonged QT interval and a flattened T wave. Early onset hypocalcemia usually presents in the first 3 days of life, and is associated with prematurity, birth asphyxia, and infants of diabetic mothers. Late onset hypocalcemia presents after the first week of life and is associated with DiGeorge syndrome, hyperphosphatemia, vitamin D deficiency, magnesium deficiency, diuretic therapy, and hypoparathyroidism. Hypocalcemia is treated with a slow infusion of calcium gluconate. Rapid infusion may cause bradycardia. Tissue infiltration with calcium causes necrosis, so administration site must be monitored.

Hypercalcemia

Hypercalcemia (>12 mg/dL) is rare, occurring less often than hypocalcemia. Signs of hypercalcemia include: Vomiting; constipation; hypertension; hypotonia; lethargy and seizures. Possible causes of hypercalcemia include: Congenital hyperparathyroidism; maternal hypoparathyroidism; hypervitaminosis D; hyperthyroidism; hypophosphatasia; subcutaneous fat necrosis; Williams syndrome; and adrenal insufficiency. Idiopathic hypercalcemia is diagnosed when no other cause can be found. Iatrogenic hypercalcemia occurs because of excess administration of calcium or vitamin D, or phosphate deprivation. Treatment depends on the exact cause, but may include:

- Correction of the underlying cause.
- Furosemide (Lasix) after adequate hydration to increase calcium excretion.
- Glucocorticoids to inhibit intestinal absorption of calcium.
- Use of low calcium and low vitamin D formulas.

Magnesium, Hypermagnesemia and Hypomagnesemia

Magnesium is the second most abundant intercellular cation:

- Neonate: 1.5-2.2 mg/dL.
- Critical values: < 1.2 mg/dL and >3 mg/dL (neonates)

Hypermagnesemia most commonly results from maternal administration of magnesium prior to delivery. Maternal serum chemistries are reflected in newborn blood values. Magnesium is used in the pregnant woman as a tocolytic agent to stop pre-term labor, and also for treatment of pre-eclampsia. Signs of hypermagnesemia in an infant include hypotonia, hyporeflexia, constipation, low blood pressure, apnea, and marked flushing secondary to vasodilatation. Elevated magnesium blocks neurosynaptic transmission by interfering with the release of acetylcholine. Treatment is usually supportive, as the elevated serum magnesium will be cleared by the infant's kidneys. In severe cases the infant may require respiratory and/or blood pressure support.

Hypomagnesemia in neonates occurs with preterm birth, respiratory distress syndrome, and neonatal hepatitis. *Symptoms* include:

- Neuromuscular excitability/ tetany.
- Seizure and coma.
- Tachycardia with ventricular arrhythmias.
- Respiratory depression.

Treatment includes diagnosing underlying cause and magnesium replacement.

Serum Potassium

Electrolyte levels in the newborn reflect those of the mother at birth. Shortly after birth (within the first 24 to 72 hours) **serum potassium** concentrations are expected to rise. This potassium rise occurs without exogenous potassium delivery and with normal renal function, and results from a shift of potassium from the intracellular space to the extracellular space. Potassium shift is more extreme in premature infants and can result in life-threatening hyperkalemia. Over the next several days, the potassium level will fall to normal in an infant with normally functioning kidneys. Preterm infants' serum electrolytes, including potassium, should be carefully monitored in the first 48 hours of life and until their values have stabilized.

Hyperkalemia

Hyperkalemia is a serum potassium level greater than 6 mEq/L in a non-hemolyzed blood sample. Squeezing the infant's heel too hard during blood collection can cause the sample to hemolyze and give an artificially elevated laboratory value. Causes of hyperkalemia in the newborn fall into 3 categories:

- Excessive potassium supplementation.
- Transcellular shift, where potassium concentrated inside cells moves outside cells, due to low pH, cellular damage, intraventricular hemorrhage or trauma.
- Decreased potassium secretion by the kidneys, due to congenital adrenal hyperplasia with elevated secretion of aldosterone or renal failure.

Cardiac manifestations of hyperkalemia include potentially fatal arrhythmias like bradycardia, tachycardia, supraventricular fibrillation, and ventricular fibrillation. EKG shows peaked T waves (earliest sign), and a widened QRS complex.

Hyperkalemia must be treated promptly because it may develop into a lethal cardiac arrhythmia, especially if the blood potassium value is >7 mEq/L and the infant's electrocardiogram shows abnormalities. Follow these steps to lower potassium levels:

- Discontinue all potassium administration.
- Elevate the blood pH by inducing hyperventilation.
- Give sodium bicarbonate to shift extracellular potassium back inside cells.
- Administer insulin and/or inhaled albuterol to enhance the shift of extracellular potassium back inside cells. *Monitor glucose levels closely.*
- Increase excretion of potassium by giving furosemide (Lasix) or sodium polystyrene sulfonate (Kayexalate).
- Give calcium gluconate concurrently to help stabilize the myocardium and lessen the chance of the infant developing an arrhythmia.
- In extreme cases, consider dialysis or exchange transfusion.

Hypokalemia

Hypokalemia is a serum potassium level less than 3.5 mEq/L. Common causes of hypokalemia are chronic diuretic use and excessive nasogastric drainage. Alkalosis accentuates hypokalemia by triggering the sequestration of potassium from the extracellular fluid to inside the cell. Electrocardiograph manifestations of hypokalemia include a flattened T wave (earliest manifestation), ST segment depression, and appearance of U waves (second recovery wave following the T wave). These changes are identical to those seen with hypomagnesemia.

Hypokalemia is usually not of concern until the level drops below 3.0 mEq/L. Signs of hypokalemia include cardiac arrhythmias, ileus, and lethargy. Treatment is with Slow-K and can be intravenous or oral. Rapid administration of potassium is associated with possible life-threatening cardiac dysfunction.

Sensible and Insensible Water Loss

Sensible water losses occur via urination, stool, and gastric drainage, and can be accurately measured. **Insensible water losses** (IWL) occur as water evaporates from the skin (2/3) or the respiratory tract (1/3). IWL cannot be directly measured. Premature neonates have thin skin that allows for increased amounts of evaporative water loss. As the skin matures and the stratum corneum develops (around 31 weeks of gestation) less water is lost through the skin. A full-term neonate will have an IWL of 12/ml/kg/24 hours at 50% humidity. Factors that increase IWL include prematurity, radiant warmers, phototherapy, fever, low humidity, and tachypnea. Infants who are mechanically ventilated should receive humidified oxygen to negate the IWL through their lungs. The NICU nurse must take into account IWL when providing fluids to neonates.

Parenteral Infusion

Most infants in the NICU require intravenous fluids, and there are a number of different types of access for **parenteral infusions**:

- Umbilical cord catheterization (arterial, venous): This is limited to a few days only.
- PICC line: This allows for long-term use without repeated IV insertions. It is particularly useful for ELBW babies although they pose the danger of thrombosis, infection, and infiltration. Percutaneous insertion sites include the saphenous, antecubital, axillary, basilic, cephalic, and external jugular veins.
- Peripheral venous access: This is used for short-term access. Extremely small catheters and introducers (Quick-cath®) may extend use to 5-7 days. There is increased risk of infiltration and skin necrosis, especially in the foot.

The catheter or needle should be secured, but must allow visualization and the site should be checked at least every hour during administration of fluids.

Volume Expanders

Volume expanders used in neonatal resuscitation include normal saline, Ringer's Lactate, and O-blood, or blood that has been cross-matched with the mother:

- Prepare 40 ml in a syringe or IV.
- Give 10 ml/kg over 5 to 10 minutes.
- Repeat if necessary.

Rapid infusion of a large volume causes intraventricular hemorrhage (5% albumin in saline is no longer the solution of choice.) Volume expanders are considered in instances where neonatal blood loss is suspected, and/or the neonate is showing signs of shock that is not responding to other resuscitative efforts. Blood loss occurs due to trauma of the placenta or umbilical cord, or with neonatal hemolysis. Shock results from inadequate tissue and organ perfusion. Signs and symptoms of shock are pallor, cold extremities, neurological depression, and weak pulses.

Metabolic acidosis

Metabolic acidosis occurs when a non-pulmonary disease or condition causes and acid-base imbalance from one of the following:

- Increased loss of bicarbonate.
- Increased production of acids.
- Decreased excretion of acids.

Blood gases will show a pH < 7.4 (acidosis) with a low bicarbonate level (<24 mmol/L) and a pCO_2 value that is **not** elevated (an elevated $PaCO_2$ would indicate a respiratory cause). Some common causes of metabolic acidosis include:

- Lactic acid production from inadequate tissue perfusion and oxygenation (asphyxia, hypoxemia, shock, severe anemia).
- Hypothermia leading to increased lactic acid production and decreased hepatic clearance of organic acids.
- Renal failure (normal kidneys reclaim bicarbonate and excrete H+ ions).
- Excessive chloride in IV fluids.
- Diarrhea, causing bicarbonate loss in stools.
- Inborn errors of metabolism that cause increased production of acids from abnormal burning of fats, proteins, or carbohydrates.

If the cause of the acidosis is metabolic, the neonate's respiratory center will be stimulated in an attempt to compensate by increasing the respiratory rate. An increased respiratory rate will decrease the serum $PaCO_2$ value and raise the blood pH (respiratory compensation). Circulating H+ ions will enter cells in exchange for potassium ions. This will blunt the lowered pH but may also cause elevated serum K+ levels, which may trigger a cardiac arrhythmia. Even though extracellular pH rises closer to normal, intracellular pH will drop, interfering with intracellular functions. The kidneys will attempt to compensate by secreting increased amounts of H+ in the urine (the urine pH is low) and conserving bicarbonate. Immature kidneys are often unable to do this efficiently, so metabolic compensation is much slower than respiratory compensation.

Metabolic Acidosis Related to High Protein/Amino Acid Feedings

Metabolic acidosis may develop in premature infants who receive high protein or amino acid feedings. The immature kidneys are unable to excrete the acids that develop as a result of protein metabolism. The NNP should screen for acidosis by checking the pH of the infant's urine. A urine pH less than 5.4 generally indicates that the kidneys are maximizing their ability to excrete acid and metabolic acidosis is present. The blood gas in this infant shows a pH < 7.4 (acidosis), a low pCO_2 level (< 40 mm/Hg) to reflect respiratory compensation, and a low bicarbonate level (< 24 mmol/L). Infants who remain in a prolonged metabolic acidotic state have less weight gain and increased excretion of sodium. Therapy with alkali or sodium chloride lessens the metabolic acidosis.

Pharmacology

Pharmacokinetics and Pharmacodynamics

Pharmacokinetics relates to the effects that the body has on a drug, and pharmacodynamics relates to the effects that a drug has on the body. Both must be considered to ensure adequate dosing to achieve the optimal response from medications. With all drugs there is an intake (dose) and a response:

Pharmacokinetics:

Pharmacokinetics relates to the route of administration, the absorption, the dosage, the frequency of administration, the distribution, and the serum levels achieved over time. The drug's rate of clearance (elimination) and doses needed to ensure therapeutic benefit must be considered. Most drugs are cleared through the kidneys, with water-soluble compounds excreted more readily than protein-soluble compounds. Volume of distribution (IV drug dose divided by plasma concentration) determines the rate at which the drug passes into tissue. Drug distribution depends on the degree of protein binding and ion trapping that takes place. Elimination halftime is the time needed to reduce plasma concentrations to 50% during elimination.

Usually the equivalent of 5 halftimes is needed to completely eliminate a drug. Five halftimes are also needed to achieve steady-state plasma concentrations if giving doses intermittently. Context-sensitive half time, in contrast, is the time needed to reach a specific amount of decrease (50%, 60%) after withdrawal of a drug. Recovery time is the length of time it takes for plasma levels to decrease to the point that the effect is eliminated. This is affected by plasma concentration. Effect-site equilibrium is the time between administration of a drug and clinical effect (the point at which the drug reaches the appropriate receptors) and must be considered when determining dose, time, and frequency of medications. The bioavailability of drugs may vary, depending upon the degree of metabolism that takes place before the drug reaches its site of action.

Pharmacodynamics

Pharmacodynamics relates to biological effects (therapeutic or adverse) of drug administration over time. Drug transport, absorption, means of elimination, and half-life must all be considered when determining effects. Responses may include continuous responses, such as blood pressure variations, or dichotomous response in which an event either occurs or does not (such as death). Information from pharmacodynamics provides feedback to modify medication dosage (pharmacokinetics). Drugs provide biological effects primarily by interacting with receptor sites (specific protein molecules) in the cell membrane. Receptors include voltage-sensitive ion channels (sodium, chloride, potassium, and calcium channels), ligand-gated ion channels, and transmembrane receptors. Agonist drugs exert effects after binding with a receptor while antagonist drugs bind with a receptor but have no effects, so they can block agonists from binding. The total number of receptors may vary, upregulating or downregulating in response to stimuli (such as drug administration). Dose-response curves show the relationship between the amount of drug given and the resultant plasma concentration and biological effects.

Drug Interactions

Drug interactions occur when one drug interferes with the activity of another in either the pharmacodynamics or pharmacokinetics:

- With *pharmacodynamic interaction,* both drugs may interact at receptor sites causing a change that results in an adverse effect or that interferes with a positive effect.
- With *pharmacokinetic interaction*, the ability of the drug to be absorbed and cleared is altered, so there may be delayed effects, changes in effects, or toxicity. Interactions may include problems in a number of areas:
  - Absorption may be increased or (more commonly) decreased, usually related to the effects within the gastrointestinal system.

- Distribution of drugs may be affected, often because of changes in protein binding.
- Metabolism may be altered, often causing changes in drug concentration.
- Biotransformation of the drug must take place, usually in the liver and gastrointestinal system, but drug interactions can impair this process.
- Clearance interactions may interfere with the body's ability to eliminate a drug, usually resulting in increased concentration of the drug.

Protein Binding

Protein binding is an important consideration for neonatal drug therapy because when drugs are bound by proteins in the blood, they are not available to be biologically active. The portion of the drug that is **not** bound to a plasma protein is the active portion. Protein binding is significant in premature neonates because they typically have:

- Lower levels of plasma proteins, such as albumin.
- Lower binding capacity.
- Susceptibility to competition from endogenous substances like bilirubin, which also attaches to plasma proteins.

Drugs that are normally highly protein bound in the adult have a higher free percentage (activity) in the neonate. Lower than expected dosages may give clinical results. Examples of drugs that are highly protein bound include Phenobarbital and Indomethacin. Is a drug with a high affinity for plasma proteins is administered, it may displace bilirubin from binding sites, increasing the neonate's risk for kernicterus.

First Pass Metabolism and Drug Clearance

First pass metabolism: This is the phenomenon that occurs to ingested drugs that are absorbed through the gastrointestinal tract and enter the hepatic portal system. Drugs metabolized on the first pass travel to the liver, where they are broken down, some to the extent that only a small fraction of the active drug circulates to the rest of the body. This first pass through the liver greatly reduces the bioavailability of some drugs. Routes of administration that avoid first pass metabolism include intravenous, intramuscular, and sublingual.

Drug Clearance: This is the ability to remove a drug from the body. The two main organs responsible for clearance are the liver and the kidneys. The liver eliminates drugs by metabolizing, or biotransforming the substance, or excreting the drug in the bile. The kidneys eliminate drugs by filtration or active excretion in the urine. Drugs use either renal or hepatic methods of clearance. Kidney and liver dysfunction inhibit the clearance of drugs that rely on that organ for removal. Toxicity results from poor clearance.

Enterohepatically Recirculated Drugs and Renally-Excreted Drugs

Enterohepatically recirculated drugs are effectively removed from circulation and then reabsorbed. These drugs are secreted in bile, which is collected in the gall bladder and emptied into the small intestine, from which part of it is reabsorbed and part excreted in the feces. This reabsorption reduces the clearance of these drugs and increases their duration of action. Generally, drugs susceptible to enterohepatic recirculation are those with a molecular weight greater than 300 g/mole and those that are amphipathic (have both a lipophilic portion and a polar portion).

Renally-excreted drugs are metabolized (biotransformed) by the liver to a form that can be excreted by the kidneys. Others are excreted by the kidneys unchanged. Infants with decreased renal function demonstrate decreased urine output or elevated levels of BUN and creatinine. The NNP should avoid using drugs that depend on the kidneys for clearance if the infant has renal impairment as overdose may result.

Formulas for Absorption, Distribution, and Clearance

Absorption: This relates to the rate at which a drug enters the blood stream and the amount of drug.

- F = the percentage of a drug's availability for absorption (with 1 equal to 100%).

Distribution: The volume of distribution is the relationship between the total loading dose of drug administered and the serum concentration. (Volume of body fluid required to dissolve the amount of drug found in the serum). This is usually expressed as units of volume per kg of weight:

- Loading dose x F = Change in concentration x volume of distribution.

Clearance: Elimination pathways (liver, kidney) can become saturated if dose of medications is too high or administration is too frequent. Ideally, a drug concentration should be maintained at a steady state (average):

- Clearance = F x Dose/dose interval x steady stage concentration.
- Dose rate = (Clearance x steady state concentration)/ F.

Principles of Administration

The half-life of a drug (t ½) is the time required to reduce serum concentrations by half, and half-life must be considered when determining **dosage and interval** of drugs for neonates. Steady state is usually achieved within 4 to 5 half-lives, and dosing interval is usually about 2-3 times the half-life. Half-life is a factor of clearance, and small or preterm infants often have reduced clearance because of slow metabolism, resulting in longer half-life. In determining dosage, the infant's weight, gestational age, as well as post-natal age must be considered. Relevant formulas include:

- T ½ = 0.7 x Volume of distribution/Clearance.
- Loading dose = (Volume of distribution x concentration)/ F.

One major problem with dosing and interval for neonates is that most drugs are not tested on infants, so about 98% are prescribed off-label. There are a number of reference tools available, including software programs, to assist with determining proper dosage and interval for neonatal medications.

Tolerance and weaning from drugs are most often concerns with administration of opiates. Tolerance occurs after repeated administration results in a lessoning of effects, requiring an increase in dosage to achieve the same results. When a neonate is weaned from a medication or a dosage is decreased, only one class of medications should be involved. Thus, if the infant is receiving both an opiate and a benzodiazepine, they should not be weaned at the same time. The infant should be evaluated for level of pain prior to weaning and the reassessed at least every 4 hours during the weaning process. Usually medications are reduced at a rate of 10% per day or 20% every other day. Infants often tolerate an initial reduction in dose better than subsequent reductions, so careful observation for signs of increased pain or withdrawal must be made. Careful control of the environment—temperature, light, and noise—should be done to reduce infant stress during the weaning process.

Routes of Medication Administration

The absorption rate of a drug depends on its transfer from its site of administration to the circulatory system. Different **routes of administration** have different absorption characteristics:

- **Oral**: Ingested medications pass from the gastrointestinal tract into the blood stream. Most absorption occurs in the small intestine and is affected by gastric motility and emptying rate, drug solubility in gastrointestinal fluids, and food presence. Orally administered drugs are susceptible to first pass metabolism by the liver.
- **Intravenous**: Medications directly administered to the blood stream have 100% absorption. Peak serum levels are rapidly achieved. Some drugs are not tolerated intravenously, due to vein irritation or toxicity, and others must be given as an infusion.
- **Intramuscular**: Medications injected into a muscle are fairly rapidly absorbed because muscle tissue is highly vascularized. Drugs in lipid vehicles absorb more slowly than those in aqueous vehicles.
- **Subcutaneous**: Medications injected beneath the skin absorb more slowly because the dermis is less vascularized than muscle. Hypoperfusion and edema decrease absorption further.

Placental Transfer of Drugs

The **placenta** acts as a barrier to protect the fetus, but its main function is to provide oxygen and nutrients for the fetus by linking the maternal and fetal circulation. Virtually all **drugs** cross the barrier to some degree, some by active transport. Some drugs are readily diffused across the placental barrier and can affect the fetus. Drugs that are non-ionized, fat-soluble and have low molecular weight diffuse easily as glucose does. Once a substance crosses the barrier, the lower pH of the fetal blood allows weakly basic drugs, such as local anesthetics and opioids, to cross into fetal circulation where they become ionized and accumulate because they can't pass back into maternal circulation (ion trapping). Giving an intravenous injection during a contraction, when uterine blood flow decreases, reduces the amount of the drug that crosses the placental barrier. A few drugs with large molecules (heparin, insulin) have minimal transfer, and lipid soluble drugs transfer more readily than water-soluble.

Relationship Between Drugs and Breastfeeding

Virtually all drugs are excreted to some degree (usually 1-2% of maternal dose) in the **breast milk**. Drugs that are highly protein-bound or have molecular weight >200 pass less easily into breast milk than lipid-soluble drugs. Breast milk is slightly acidic compared to plasma, so compounds that are weakly alkaline may be present in breast milk in larger amounts than in plasma. Mothers should be advised to take medications after breastfeeding to minimize transfer. Some medications have adverse effects on infants:

- **Opiates:** Sedation.
- **Aspirin**: Risk of Reye's syndrome.
- **Antibiotics**: Penicillins may cause diarrhea; tetracycline, stained/mottled teeth, and chloramphenicol, gray baby syndrome.
- **Antifungals**: GI symptoms, such as diarrhea, vomiting; blood dyscrasias.
- **Cardiovascular drugs:** Reserpine may cause diarrhea, bradycardia, lethargy, and respiratory distress; propanolol may cause respiratory depression, bradycardia, or hypoglycemia.

- **Psychotherapeutic agents:** Sedation, poor feeding. Lithium may cause cyanosis and hypoventilation.
- **Ethanol:** Lethargy, drowsiness, depressed motor development.

Acetaminophen

Acetaminophen (Tylenol®) is used both for control of mild to moderate pain and fever. Acetaminophen can be administered orally and rectally, but absorption is less reliable with the rectal route. Acetaminophen has a half-life of 4 hours and is conjugated in the liver and excreted renally. Oral dosage is typically 24 mg/kg as a loading dose and 12 mg/kg every four hours (or 8 hours in infants <32 weeks gestation), and rectal dosage 36 mg/kg (loading) followed by 24 mg/kg every 8 hours. Serum levels should be checked if treatment is to continue for >24 hours. Serum levels of 12-24 mg/L are required for adequate pain control. Acetaminophen is commonly used for control of pain after circumcision although it is not sufficient for pain control during the procedure.

Analgesics/Narcotics

Fentanyl and morphine are opioid **analgesics/narcotics** that treat moderate to severe pain.

- **Fentanyl** is for painful dressing changes or procedures. Duration of action is 1-2 hours and half-life is 2-4 hours. Dosage is 1-4 micrograms/kg every 1-2 hours or by continuous infusion. Rapid tolerance develops, requiring higher doses to create the same relief, and increasing the chance of overdose. Fentanyl is metabolized by the liver and excreted by the kidneys. Side effects of fentanyl include: Respiratory depression; peripheral vasodilatation; inhibition of intestinal peristalsis; and chest wall rigidity at higher doses, compromising ventilation. Fentanyl is less likely to cause hypotension than morphine.
- **Morphine** is for post-operative pain. Duration of action is 3-4 hours and half-life is 2-4 hours. Morphine is metabolized by the liver to an inactive metabolite and excreted by the kidneys; 2-12% is excreted unchanged in the urine. Dosage is 0.02 to 0.1 mg/kg every 1-4 hours or by continuous infusion. Side effects of morphine include: Respiratory depression, histamine release, and seizures.

Anticoagulants

Neonates may require **anticoagulant therapy** for thrombosis, sometimes associated with catheters used for critical care or thrombocytosis associated with iron-deficiency anemia. Anticoagulant therapy poses fewer risks than fibrinolytic therapy although excessive bleeding may occur. Anticoagulants include:

- Unfractionated heparin:
  - Preterm infants: Initial bolus of 50 units/kg and maintenance of 15 units to 35 units/kg/hr to maintain level of 0.3 to 0.7 units/mL.
  - Full-term infants: Initial bolus of 100 units/kg and maintenance of 25 units to 50 units/kg/hr to maintain level of 0.3 to 0.7 unit/mL.
- Low-molecular-weight heparin: 1.7 mg/kg sq every 12 hours or as needed to maintain level of 0.5 to 1 units/ml 4 hours after administration.
- Warfarin: May be used in rare cases, such as genetic deficiencies of protein C or S (purpura fulminans), for long-term therapy.

Infants that are heparin resistant may be administered fresh frozen plasma (1 mL/kg every 24-48 hours) or AT concentrate (50-150 units/kg every 24-48 hours) to enhance effect of heparin.

Anticonvulsants

Anticonvulsants are used to treat seizures, which often indicate central nervous system dysfunction. Seizures are more common during the neonatal period than later in infancy/childhood and are associated with low birth weight. Treatment is critical to prevent brain damage, but drugs may cause sedation, rash, and blood dyscrasias:

- **Phenobarbital** (Luminal®) is the neonatal drug of choice. Loading dose is 20 mg/kg IV in 10-15 minutes and then 5 mg/kg to maximum 40 mg/kg to control seizures. Maintenance dose is 3 to 4 mg /kg/24 hours in 2 doses beginning ≥12 hours after loading dose. Infant should be provided oxygen and ventilation as needed.
- **Fosphenytoin** (Cerbxy®) is used if phenobarbitalis ineffective. It has high water solubility and neutral pH and does not cause tissue injury. It can be administered IV or IM. Loading dose is 15 to 20mgPE/kg and maintenance id 4 to 8mg PE/kg/24 hrs. Blood pressure should be monitored and caution exercised with hyperbilirubinemia.
- **Phenytoin** (Dilantin®) is sometimes used instead of fosphenytoin if phenobarbital is ineffective. It is incompatible with other drugs and glucose and can cause hypotension, bradycardia, and dysrhythmias if administered too quickly and cannot be given IM or in central lines. Loading dose is 15-20 mg/kg IV over 30 minutes, and maintenance is 4-8 mg/kg/24 hours. Line must be flushed with NS.
- **Lorazepam** (Ativan®) is used if other drugs are ineffective in controlling seizures. Onset is action is very rapid (<5 minutes), so the infant must be monitored carefully for respiratory depression. Medication is administered by slow IV push over a number of minutes at 0.05 to 0.1 mg/kg.

In some cases, seizures are triggered by hypoglycemia, and treatment includes glucose 10% solution. Pyridoxine (B_6) deficiency may also cause seizures and is treated with IV or IM Vitamin B_6.

Antimicrobials and Antibiotics

Antimicrobials include antibiotics, antifungals, and antivirals.

Antibiotics may be classified according to their chemical nature, origin, action, or range of effectiveness. Broad-spectrum antibiotics are useful against both Gram-positive and Gram-negative bacteria. Medium spectrum antibiotics are usually effective against Gram-positive bacteria although some may also be effective against Gram-negative. Narrow spectrum antibiotics are effective against a small range of bacteria. Antibiotics function by killing the bacteria by interfering with its biological functions (bacteriocidal) or by preventing reproduction (bacteriostatic).

Gentamicin

Gentamicin is an inexpensive aminoglycosides antibiotic commonly used to treat neonates with Gram-negative bacterial infections, like *Staphylococci*. It works by interfering with bacterial protein synthesis, resulting in a defective bacterial cell membrane. Gentamicin is excreted unmetabolized by the kidneys and renal function is directly related to clearance. Clearance is slower in premature neonates secondary to immature kidneys. The peak level (highest concentration in the blood) of gentamicin is measured 30 minutes after infusion is completed and trough level (lowest concentration of the drug in the blood) is measured 30 minutes prior to the next dose. Potential toxicities from elevated gentamicin levels are ototoxity (ear damage potentiated by concurrent use of furosemide) and nephrotoxicity (kidney damage), so patients with renal failure may only require dosing once every several days. If the pre-dose level falls below 0.5 mg/L and the post dose level falls below 4 mg/L, the gentamicin is sub-therapeutic and will not kill the bacterial infection.

Vaccinations

There are a number of different types of **vaccines**:

- **Conjugated forms:** An organism is altered and then joined (conjugated) with another substance, such as a protein, to potentiate immune response (such as conjugated Hib).
- **Killed virus vaccines:** The virus has been killed but can still cause an immune response (such as inactivated poliovirus).
- **Live virus vaccines:** The virus is live but in a weakened (attenuated) form so that it doesn't cause the disease but confers immunity (such as measles vaccine).
- **Recombinant forms:** The organism is genetically altered and for example, may use proteins rather than the whole cell to stimulate immunity (such as Hepatitis B and acellular pertussis vaccine).
- **Toxoid**: A toxin (antigen) that has been weakened by the use of heat or chemicals so it is too weak to cause disease but stimulates antibodies.

Some vaccines are given shortly after birth; others begin at 2 months, 12 months, or 2 years and some later in childhood.

Hepatitis B Vaccine

Hepatitis B is transmitted through blood and body fluids, including during birth; therefore, it is now recommended for all newborns as well as all those<18 and those in high risk groups >18 (drug users, men having sex with men, those with multiple sex partners, partners of those with HBV, and healthcare workers). Hepatitis B can cause serious liver disease leading to liver cancer. Three injections of monovalent HepB are required to confer immunity:

- Birth (within 12 hours).
- Between 1-2 months.
- ≥24 weeks.

Note: If combination vaccines are given after the birth dose then a dose at 4 months can be given.

If the mother is Hepatitis B positive, the child should be given both the monovalent HepB vaccination as well as HepB immune globulin within 12 hours of birth. Adverse reactions include local irritation and fever. Severe allergic reactions can occur to those allergic to baker's yeast.

Inactivated Poliovirus Vaccine

Poliomyelitis is a serious viral infection that can cause paralysis and death. Prior to introduction of a vaccine in 1955, polio was responsible for >20,000 cases in the United States each year. There have been no cases of polio caused by the poliovirus for >20 years in the United States, but it still occurs in some third world countries, so continuing vaccinations is very important. Oral polio vaccine (OPV) is no longer recommended in the United States because it carries a very slight risk of causing the disease (1:2.4 million). Children require 4 doses of injectable polio vaccine (IPV):

- 2 months
- 4 months
- 6-18 months
- 4-6 years (booster dose)

IPV is contraindicated for those who have had a severe reaction to neomycin, streptomycin, or polymyxin B. Rare allergic reactions can occur, but there are almost no serious problems caused by this vaccine.

Diphtheria, Tetanus, and Pertussis Vaccine and Rotavirus Vaccine

Diphtheria and pertussis (whooping cough) are highly contagious bacterial diseases of the upper respiratory tract. Cases of diphtheria are now rare; however, recent outbreaks of pertussis have occurred in the United States. Tetanus is a bacterial infection contracted through cuts, wounds, and scratches. The **diphtheria, tetanus, and pertussis (DTaP) vaccine** is recommended for all children. DTaP requires 5 doses:

- 2 months
- 4 months
- 6 months
- 5-18 months
- 4-6 years (or at 11-12 years if booster missed between 4-6)

Rotavirus is a cause of significant morbidity and mortality in children, especially in developing countries, but most children, without vaccination, will suffer from severe diarrhea caused by rotavirus within the first 5 years of life. The new rotavirus vaccine is advised for all infants but should not be initiated after 12 weeks or administered after 32 weeks, so there is a narrow window of opportunity. Three doses are required:

- 2 months (between 6-12 weeks)
- 4 months
- 6 months

Heptavalent Pneumococcal Conjugate Vaccine and Haemophilus Influenzae Type B Vaccine

Heptavalent pneumococcal conjugate vaccine (PCV-7) (Prevnar®) was released for use in the United States in 2001 for treatment of children under 2 years old. It provides immunity to 7 serotypes of *Streptococcus pneumoniae* to protect against invasive pneumococcal disease, such as pneumonia, otitis media, bacteremia, and meningitis. Because children are most at risk ≥1, vaccinations begin early:

Administration:
- 1st dose: 6-8 weeks
- 2nd dose: 4 months
- 3rd dose: 6 months
- 4th dose: 12-18 months.

***Haemophilus influenzae* type B (HIB) vaccine** (HibTITER® and PedavaxHIB®) protects against infection with *Haemophilus influenzae,* which can cause serious respiratory infections, pneumonia, meningitis, bacteremia, and pericarditis in children ≥5 years old. *Administration:*

- 1st dose: 2 months
- 2nd dose: 4 months
- 3rd dose: 6 months (may be required, depending upon the brand of vaccine)
- Last dose: 12-15 months (this booster dose must be given at least 2 months after the earlier doses for those who start at a later age than 2 months.

Anti-Hypertensives and Other Cardiac Drugs

Antihypertensives are used to control congestive heart failure and reduce the cardiac workload:

- **Captopril** is an ace inhibitor is used to control hypertension.
- **Propranolol** is a beta-blocker used to control hypertension.
- **Labetalol** (Normodyne®, Trandate®) is an alpha-1 and beta-adrenergic blocker that slows the heart rate and decreases peripheral vascular resistance and cardiac output.

Miscellaneous cardiac drugs are used for specific purposes:

- **Calcium chloride/Calcium gluconate** is given intravenously after surgery to increase myocardial contractibility.
- **Brevibloc** (Esmolol®) is a beta-blocker given intravenously after surgery to control systemic hypertension, arrhythmias, and outflow obstruction.
- **Indomethacin** (Indocin®) is a NSAID that is given intravenously to inhibit the production of prostaglandin, thereby speeding the closure of the ductus arteriosus.
- **Prostaglandin** is given intravenously before surgery to maintain the patency of the ductus arteriosus for structural cardiac abnormalities in conditions such as coarctation of the aorta or transposition of the great arteries.

Diuretics Used for Infants with Cardiac Disease/Abnormalities

Diuretics are used in the cardiac patient to increase renal perfusion and filtration, thereby reducing preload. Dosages are weight and age related. Diuretics commonly used include:

- **Bumetanide** (Bumex®) is a loop diuretic (acting on the renal ascending loop of Henle) given intravenously after surgery to reduce preload.
- **Ethacrynic acid** (Edecrin®) is a loop diuretic given intravenously after surgery to reduce preload.
- **Furosemide** (Lasix®) is a loop diuretic and is used for the control of congestive heart failure as well as renal insufficiency. It is used after surgery to decrease preload and to reduce the inflammatory response caused by cardiopulmonary bypass (post-perfusion syndrome).
- **Spironolactone** (Aldactone®) is a potassium-sparing synthetic steroid diuretic that increases the secretion of both water and sodium and is used to treat congestive heart failure. It may be given orally or intravenously.

Loop, Thiazide, and Potassium-Sparing Diuretics

Diuretics decrease the fluid load in infants with heart failure or lung disorders, such as bronchopulmonary dysplasia. Different classes of diuretics have different mechanisms of action and different side effect profiles:

- **Loop diuretics** (e.g., furosemide) are the most potent of the diuretics and work on the ascending limb of the loop of Henle. They disrupt the $Na+/K+/2Cl-$ transporter and also limit $K+$ reabsorption. Hypokalemia, hyponatremia, and increased calcium excretion are the adverse reactions seen with chronic use.
- **Thiazide diuretics** (e.g., chlorothiazide) work by inhibiting $Na+/Cl-$ transport in the distal convoluted tubule. They are less potent than loop diuretics. Hyponatremia, hypokalemia, and hypomagnesemia are the adverse reactions from chronic use.

- 106 -

- *Potassium-sparing diuretics* (e.g., spironolactone) work by inhibiting the action of aldosterone. Aldosterone promotes K+ secretion and Na+ reabsorption at the distal nephron. These diuretics are the least potent, but do not cause hypokalemia.

Vasodilators and Anti-Arrhythmics

Vasodilators may be used for arterial dilation or venous dilation. These drugs are used to treat pulmonary hypertension or generalized systemic hypertension. Dosages are weight and age related. Vasodilators include:

- *Nitroglycerine* is used intravenously after surgery to improve myocardial perfusion by dilating the coronary arteries. It can be used as a venous dilator and decreases the diastolic pressure of the left ventricle and reduces systemic vascular resistance (SVR).
- *Nitroprusside* is given intravenously before and after surgery for peripheral vascular dilation to decrease afterload and SVR in order to increase cardiac output.

Anti-arrhythmics are used to control arrhythmias and slow the heart rate.

- *Amiodarone* is given intravenously after surgery to reduce AV and SA conduction, slowing the heartbeat. It is used to control both ventricular dysrhythmias and junctional ectopic tachycardia.
- *Lidocaine* is given intravenously before and after surgery to control ventricular dysrhythmias.
- *Procainamide* is given intravenously after surgery to control supraventricular tachycardia and is effective for both atrial and ventricular tachycardia.

Vasopressors/Inotropes

Drugs used to increase cardiac output and improve contractibility of the myocardium are the **vasopressors/inotropes**. Dosage and administration of pediatric medications is weight and age related. Inotropes include:

- *Dobutamine* is given intravenously before and after surgery to improve cardiac output and treat cardiac decompensation.
- *Dopamine* is given intravenously before and after surgery to increase cardiac output, blood pressure, and the excretion of urine.
- *Digoxin* is given intravenously or by mouth and is used to increase the strength of myocardial contractions, resulting in better cardiac output.
- *Epinephrine* is given intravenously before and after surgery to increase blood pressure and cardiac output, but it must be used judiciously because it also increases consumption of oxygen.
- *Milrinone/Amrinone* is given after surgery to increase cardiac output and stroke volume, decrease systemic vascular resistance (SVR) as well as control congestive heart failure.

Digitalis

Digitalis is a cardiac glycoside that is used to treat congestive heart failure (CHF) and several different cardiac arrhythmias. Digitalis slows and strengthens the heartbeat. It has both a direct action on the myocardium and an indirect action mediated through the autonomic nervous system. The direct effect on the myocardium works by inhibiting the action of the sodium/potassium pump across cardiac cell membranes. The net result is an increase in intracellular sodium and calcium

- 107 -

and an increase in extracellular potassium. The intracellular calcium is responsible for the increased strength of contractions of the heart (positive ionotrope). The indirect action of digitalis causes the heart rate to slow (negative chronotrope) by decreasing electrical conduction through the AV node. Digoxin has a narrow therapeutic index, meaning the lethal dose is close to the therapeutic dose. Signs of digitalis toxicity in infants include:

- GI signs: Anorexia, nausea, vomiting, and diarrhea.
- Cardiac arrhythmias: Most commonly conduction disturbances, such as first-degree heart block, a supraventricular tachyarrhythmia such as atrial tachycardia, or bradycardia.

Volatile Anesthetics

Small infants have a high water content (70-75%) compared to adults (50-60%), and a lower muscle mass. These factors, coupled with slow renal and hepatic clearance, increased rate of metabolism, decreased protein binding, and increased organ perfusion affect the pharmacological action of drugs. Pediatric doses are calculated according to the child's weight in kilograms, but other factors may affect dosage. **Anesthetic agents** must be chosen with care because of the potential for adverse effects:

- ***Inhalational***: Infants are more likely to develop hypotension and bradycardia with inhalational anesthetic agents. Inhalation induction is rapid because infants and young children have high alveolar ventilation and decreased FRC compared to older patients with depression of ventilation more common in infants. There is increased risk of overdose. Sevoflurane is usually preferred for induction and isoflurane or halothane for maintenance as desflurane and sevoflurane are associated with delirium on emergence.

Nonvolatile Anesthetics

Pediatric **anesthetic agents** include:

- ***Nonvolatile***: Infants may need higher proportionate (based on weight) doses of *propofol* because it is eliminated more quickly than with adults. It should not be used for infants who are critically ill, as it has been correlated to increased mortality rate and severe adverse effects leading to multi-organ failure. *Thiopental* also is used in higher proportionate doses for infants and children although this is not true for neonates. Neonates are especially sensitive to opioids, and *morphine* should be avoided or used with caution. Clearance rates for some drugs (sufentanil, alfentanil) may be higher in infants. *Ketamine* combined with *fentanyl* may cause more hypotension in neonates and small infants than ketamine combined with midazolam. *Midazolam* combined with fentanyl can cause severe hypotension. *Etomidate* is not used for infants but is reserved for children >10.

Muscle Relaxants/Paralytics

Pediatric **anesthetic agents** include:

- **Muscle relaxants:** Onset with muscle relaxants is about 50% shorter in infants than adults, and pediatric patients may have variable responses to muscle to non-depolarizing muscle relaxants. Drugs that are metabolized through the liver (pancuronium, vecuronium, and cisatracurium) have prolonged action, so atracurium and cisatracurium, which do not depend on the liver, are more reliable. Succinylcholine can cause severe adverse effects (rhabdomyolysis, malignant hyperthermia, hyperkalemia, arrhythmias), so its use requires premedication with atropine, but succinylcholine is usually avoided in pediatric patients except for rapid sequence induction for children with full stomach and laryngospasm. Rocuronium is frequently used for intubation because of fast onset, but it has up to 90 minutes duration, so mivacurium, atracurium, and cisatracurium may be preferred for shorter procedures. Nerve stimulators should be used to monitor incremental doses, which are usually 25-30% of the original bolus. Blockade by non-depolarizing muscle relaxants can be reversed with neostigmine or edrophonium and glycopyrrolate or atropine.

Bronchodilators and Respiratory Stimulants

Bronchodilators and respiratory stimulants are used to treat respiratory distress in the neonate:

- **Aminophylline and theophylline** both stimulate the sympathetic nervous system and dilate the bronchi. These medications are used for apnea of prematurity in the neonate and bronchospasm in infants with respiratory distress. Apnea of prematurity is treated with loading dose of 6 mg/kg aminophylline with maintenance doses of 2.5-3.5 mg/kg intravenously every 12 hours. Further treatment may be done orally with theophylline. Side effects include tachycardia, seizures, and irritability.
- **Albuterol** is a selective $\beta2$-adrenergic agonist bronchodilator that can be administered orally (100-300 µg/kg 3-4 times daily) or inhaled (100-500 µg/kg 4-8 times daily).
- **Caffeine citrate,** a stimulant, is the first line treatment for apnea of prematurity as it is safer than theophylline and can be administered orally. Loading dose is usually 20 mg/mg with one-time daily maintenance dose of 5mg/kg.
- **Epinephrine** is used to treat stridor with effect on β-adrenoreceptors. It is delivered with nebulizer at 50-100 µg/kg as needed.

Surfactants

Surfactants reduce surface tension to prevent collapse of alveoli. Beractant (Survanta®) is derived from bovine lung tissue and calfactant (Infasurf®) from calf lung tissue. Surfactant replacement therapy is used to prevent RDS for infants born at 27-30 weeks gestation. It is also used for infants showing signs of worsening lung disease. Surfactant is given via the endotracheal tube (ETT) as an inhalant. All four lung fields are coated with surfactant, so the dose is roughly divided into four equal parts. The head of the bed is declined to put the baby in a head down position. The head is turned to one direction, and the first dose is put down the ETT. To reach the other upper lung field, the head is turned the other direction, and the second dose given vial the ETT. Once the upper lung fields have received their doses, the head of the bed is inclined to reach the lower fields. The head turning procedure is repeated until all four doses have been given.

Inhaled Nitrous Oxide (iNO)

Inhaled nitrous oxide (iNO), a selective pulmonary vasodilator, is used to treat persistent pulmonary hypertension of the newborn in neonates without congenital heart disease and with mean airway pressure of 12-15 cm H_2O, decreased PaO_2, and pH >7.40 despite treatments and adequate ventilation. Treatment with conventional therapy (such as pressor/inotropics) should continue. ***Protocols*** may differ somewhat:

- iNO is initiated at 40 ppm NO for 1 hour and increased to 80 ppm for an additional hour if the PaO_2 does not improve.
- When PaO_2 reaches 70 mm Hg, the iNO can be decreased to 40 ppm.
- If PaO_2 reaches and stays at 100-150 mm Hg, the iNO should be decreased to 20 ppm and then to 10 ppm in 24 hours if the level maintains.
- If the PaO_2 decreases to below 60 mm Hg, the iNO should be increased to previous dosage.
- Abrupt discontinuation must be avoided as it may cause rebound increase peripheral vascular resistance.

Note: iNO combines with hemoglobin, which inactivates the NO and forms methemoglobin, so methemoglobin levels must be monitored at 1, 2, and 4 hours after initiating therapy and then every 6 to 8 hours when receiving ≥40 ppm or every 12 hours if receiving <40 ppm.

Respiratory Stimulants

Respiratory stimulants are medications used to stimulate respirations in infants with apnea or prematurity or other causes of apnea.

Caffeine	IV/PO: 10-20 mg/kg and then 5-10 mg/kg daily for maintenance.	Drug of choice for treatment of apnea of prematurity, may be used for apnea after extubation or ventilation. May result in decreased incidence of bronchopulmonary dysplasia with VLBW. May cause GI upset, vomiting, bloody stools.
Theophylline	IV/PO: 4-5 mg/kg and then 3-6 mg/kg/d for maintenance. *NOTE*: If aminophylline used, dosage should be increased by 20-25%.	For treatment of apnea of prematurity, may be for apnea after extubation or ventilation and with prostaglandin E1 (used to treat heart defects). May cause tachycardia, vomiting, and hyperglycemia.
Doxapram	IV: 1-2 mg/kg/hr. PO: 12-24 mg/kg every 6 hours.	May cause decreased cerebral blood flow so should be avoided unless other treatments ineffective.

Hypnotics

Hypnotics include barbiturate drugs and benzodiazepines, and may be used to help relieve pain or seizures and for neonates on ventilation that are receiving neuromuscular blockers. Neonates must be monitored for excessive sedation and respiratory depression. Commonly used hypnotics include:

Lorazepam	IV/PO: 0.05 to 0.1 mg/kg every 1-2 hours as needed.	May be used to treat seizures and for sedation. May contain benz alcohol.

Phenobarbital	IV/PO 2.5mg/kg twice daily.	Used for neonatal abstinence syndrome but rarely for sedation because of rapid development of tolerance.
Midazolam	IV 0.05-0.25 mg/kg every 2-4 hours. PO 0.25 mg/kg or Intranasal 0.3 mg/kg: 30-60 minutes pre-procedure.	Contains benzyl alcohol. Neonates should not receive more than 25mg/kg of benzyl alcohol per day.
Dexmede-tomidine	IV: 0.25-1 mcg/kg/hour.	Start at low dose and increase in increments of 0.25 mcg/kg/hr every 2 to 4 hours. Requires weaning at rate of 0.1 mcg/kg/hr every 12 to 48 hours. If neonate has received drug for more than 3 days, oral clonidine may be given during weaning.

Steroids

Steroids are commonly administered to mothers to promote fetal lung development for preterm births. These drugs include betamethasone and dexamethasone. Steroids may also be administered to the neonate, but they are associated with significant side effects:

- *Betamethasone* may be used for chronic lung disease (CLD) in the neonate and post-intubation airway edema, but high dose treatment has been associated with cerebral palsy, growth depression, hypertension, hyperglycemia, hypokalemia, and increased risk of infection. Airway edema is treated with 200 µg/kg orally/IV every 8 hours beginning 4 hours before extubation. Dosages for other treatment vary widely with tapering of doses.
- *Hydrocortisone* may be used for physiologic replacement or acute hypotension. Replacement is begun with 1-2 mg orally every 8 hours and increased to 6-9 mg/m2/day. Hypotension is treated with 2 mg/kg IV loading dose and maintenance of 1 mg/kg IV every 8-12 hours

Gastrointestinal Drugs

Gastrointestinal drugs used to treat gastroesophageal reflux and to reduce gastric acid include:

Antacids (calcium and aluminum containing)	PO: 50-150 mg/kg/day in divided doses every 4 to 6 hours (aluminum hydroxide).	Although antacids reduce gastric acid and promote healing of the esophagus, they are not commonly used because they cause constipation in the neonate and may increase risk of fractures later in life
Prokinetic agents (metoclopramide)	PO: 0.1 to 0.15 mg/kg every 8 to 12 hours.	Increase gastric motility. Sometimes used for feeding intolerance. Complications may include dystonic reaction.
Proton Pump inhibitors (omeprazole)	PO: 0.5 to 1.5 mg/kg daily for ≤8 weeks.	Reduce production of gastric acid, but may increase risk of fracture later in life. May be used for refractory duodenal ulcer or reflux esophagitis.

The Disease Process

Cardiac

Cyanotic and Acyanotic Congenital Cardiac Defects

Congenital heart disease is one of the leading causes of death in children within the first year of life. There are two main types of congenital heart disease: acyanotic and cyanotic. They may also be classified according to hemodynamics related to the blood flow pattern.

Cyanotic congenital heart disease includes those with decreased pulmonary blood flow and mixed blood flow.

Decreased pulmonary blood flow	Tetralogy of Fallot
	Tricuspid atresia
Mixed blood flow	Ebstein's anomaly
	Hypoplastic left heart syndrome
	Total anomalous pulmonary venous return
	Transposition of great arteries
	Truncus arteriosus

Acyanotic defects include those with increased pulmonary blood flow or obstructed ventricular blood flow.

Increased pulmonary blood flow	Atrial septal defect
	Atrioventricular canal defect
	Patent ductus arteriosus
	Ventricular septal defect
Obstructed ventricular blood flow	Aortic stenosis
	Coarctation of aorta
	Pulmonic stenosis

Ebstein's Anomaly

Ebstein's anomaly is an abnormality of the tricuspid valve separating the right atrium from the right ventricle with the valve leaflets displaced downward and one adhering to the wall so that there is backflow into the atrium when the ventricle contracts. This usually results in enlargement of the right atrium and congestive heart failure. As pressure increases in the right atrium, it usually forces the foramen ovale to stay open so that the blood is shunted to the left atrium, mixing the deoxygenated blood with oxygenated blood that then leaves through the aorta. Symptoms vary widely depending upon the degree of defect and range from asymptomatic to life threatening. Many children are not diagnosed until their teens.

Symptoms include:

- Cyanosis with low oxygen saturation.
- Congestive heart failure.
- Palpitations, arrhythmias.
- Dyspnea on exertion.
- Increased risk for bacterial endocarditis.

Treatment:

- ACE inhibitors, diuretics, and digoxin.
- Surgical repair of abnormalities with valve repair or replacement.

Tetralogy of Fallot

Tetralogy of Fallot (TOF) is a combination of 4 different defects:

- **Ventricular septal defect** (usually with a large opening).
- **Pulmonic stenosis** with decreased blood flow to lungs.
- **Overriding aorta** (displacement to the right so that it appears to come from both ventricles, usually overriding the ventricular septal defect), resulting in mixing of oxygenated and deoxygenated blood.
- Right ventricular hypertrophy.

Infants are often acutely cyanotic immediately after birth while others with less severe defects may have increasing cyanosis over the first year. *Symptoms* include:

- Intolerance to feeding or crying, resulting in increased cyanotic "blue spells" or "tet spells."
- Failure to thrive with poor growth.
- Clubbing of fingers may occur over time.
- Intolerance to activity as child grows.
- Increased risk for emboli, brain attacks, brain abscess, seizures, fainting or sudden death.

Treatment: Total surgical repair at ≥1 year is now the preferred treatment rather than palliative procedures formerly used.

Truncus Arteriosus

Truncus arteriosus is the blood from both ventricles flowing into one large artery with one valve, with more blood flowing to the lower pressure pulmonary arteries than to the body, resulting in low oxygen saturation and hypoxemia. Usually, there is a ventricular septal defect so the blood in the ventricles mixes.

Symptoms include:

- Congestive heart failure with pulmonary edema because of increased blood flow to lungs.
- Typical symptoms of congestive heart failure.
- Cyanosis, especially about the face (mouth and nose).
- Dyspnea, increasing on feeding or exertion.
- Poor feeding and failure to thrive.
- Heart murmur.
- Increased risk for brain abscess and bacterial endocarditis.

Treatment includes:

- Palliative banding of the pulmonary arteries to decrease the flow of blood to the lungs.
- Surgical repair with cardiopulmonary bypass includes closing the ventricular defect, utilizing the existing single artery as the aorta by separating the pulmonary arteries from it and creating a conduit between the pulmonary arteries and the right ventricle.

Transposition of Great Arteries

Transposition of great arteries is the aorta and pulmonary artery arising from the wrong ventricle (aorta from the right ventricle and pulmonary artery from the left), so there is no connection between pulmonary and systemic circulation with deoxygenated blood being pumped back to the body and the oxygenated blood from the lungs is pumped back to the lungs. Septal defects may also occur, allowing some mixing of blood and the ductus arteriosus allows mixing until it closes. *Symptoms* vary depending upon whether there is mixing of blood but may include:

- Mild to severe cyanosis.
- Symptoms of congestive heart failure.
- Cardiomegaly develops in the weeks after birth.
- Heart sounds vary depending upon the severity of the defects.

Treatment may include:

- Prostaglandin to keep the ductus arteriosus and foramen ovale open. Balloon atrial septostomy to increase size of foramen ovale.
- Surgical repair to transpose arteries to the normal position ("arterial switch") as well of repair septal defects and other abnormalities.

Total Anomalous Pulmonary Venous Return

Total anomalous pulmonary venous return is a defect in which the 4 pulmonary veins connect to the right atrium by an anomalous connection rather than the right atrium so there is no direct blood flow to the left side of the heart; however, an atrial septal defect is common and allows for the mixed oxygenated and deoxygenated blood to shunt to the left and enter the aorta. There are 4 different types of anomalies, and in some cases pulmonary vein obstruction. If the pulmonary veins are not obstructed, children may be asymptomatic initially.

Symptoms include:

- Heart murmur.
- Severe post-natal cyanosis or mild cyanosis.
- Dyspnea with grunting and sternal retraction or dyspnea on exertion.
- Low oxygen saturation (in the 80s if there is no pulmonary obstruction).
- Cardiomegaly (right-sided hypertrophy).

Treatment includes:

- Surgical repair to attach the pulmonary veins to the left atrium and correct any other defects may be done immediately after birth or delayed for 1-2 months.

Tricuspid Atresia

Tricuspid atresia is lack of tricuspid valve between the right atrium and right ventricle so blood flows through the foramen ovale or an atrial defect to the left atrium and then through a ventricular wall defect from the left ventricle to the right ventricle and out to the lungs, causing oxygenated and deoxygenated bloods to mix. Pulmonic obstruction is common.

Symptoms include:

- Postnatal cyanosis obvious.
- Tachycardia and dyspnea.
- Increasing hypoxemia and clubbing in older children.
- Increased risk for bacterial endocarditis, brain abscess, and brain attack.

Treatment includes:

- Prostaglandin (alprostadil), to keep the ductus arteriosus and foramen ovale open if there are no septal defects.
- Numerous surgical procedures, including pulmonary artery banding, shunting from the aorta to the pulmonary arteries, Glenn procedure (connecting superior vena cava to pulmonary artery to allow deoxygenated blood to flow to the lungs), atrial septostomy to enlarge the opening between the atria, and the Fontan corrective procedure (usually done at 2-4 years after previous stabilizing procedures).

Patent Ductus Arteriosus

Patent ductus arteriosus (PDA) is failure of the ductus arteriosus that connects the pulmonary artery and aorta to close after birth, resulting in left to right shunting of blood from the aorta back to the pulmonary artery. This increases the blood flow to the lung and causes an increase in pulmonary hypertension that can result in damage to the lung tissue.

Symptoms include:

- Essentially asymptomatic (some infants).
- Cyanosis.
- Congestive heart failure.
- Machinery-like murmur.
- Frequent respiratory infections and dyspnea, especially on exertion.
- Widened pulse pressure.
- Bounding pulse.
- Atrial fibrillation/palpitations.
- Increased risk for bacterial endocarditis, congestive heart failure, and development of pulmonary vascular obstructive disease.

Treatment includes:

- Indomethacin (Indocin®) given within 10 days of birth is successful in closing about 80% of defects.
- Surgical repair with ligation of the patent vessel.

Ventricular Septal Defect (VSD)

Ventricular septal defect (VSD) is an abnormal opening in the septum between the right and left ventricles. If the opening is small, the child may be asymptomatic, but larger openings can result in a left to right shunt because of higher pressure in the left ventricle. This shunting increases over 6 weeks after birth with symptoms becoming more evident, but the defect may close within a few years.

Symptoms may include:

- Congestive heart failure with peripheral edema.
- Tachycardia.
- Dyspnea.
- Difficulty feeding.
- Heart murmur.
- Recurrent pulmonary infections.
- Increased risk for bacterial endocarditis and pulmonary vascular obstructive disease.

Treatment includes:

- Diuretics, such as furosemide (Lasix®) may be used for congestive heart failure.
- ACE inhibitor (Captopril®) to decrease pulmonary hypertension.
- Surgical repair includes pulmonary banding or cardiopulmonary bypass repair of the opening with suturing or a patch, depending upon the size.

Coarctation of the Aorta

Coarctation of the aorta is a stricture of the aorta, proximal to the ductus arteriosus intersection. The increased blood pressure caused by the heart attempting to pump the blood past the stricture causes the heart to enlarge and also blood pressure to the head and upper extremities while decreasing blood pressure and to the lower body and extremities. With severe stricture, symptoms may not occur until the ductus arteriosus closes, causing sudden loss of blood supply to the lower body.

Symptoms include:

- Difference in blood pressure between upper and lower extremities.
- Congestive heart failure symptoms in infants.
- Headaches, dizziness, and nosebleeds in older children.
- Increased risk of hypertension, ruptured aorta, aortic aneurysm, bacterial endocarditis, and brain attack.

Treatment includes:

- Prostaglandin (alprostadil), such as Prostin VR Pediatric®, to reopen the ductus arteriosus for infants.
- Balloon angioplasty.
- Surgical resection and anastomosis or graft replacement (usually at 3-5 years of age unless condition is severe). Infants who have surgery may need later repair.

Atrial Septal Defect (ASD)

An **atrial septal defect (ASD)** is an abnormal opening in the septum between the right and left atria. Because the left atrium has higher pressure than the right atrium, some of the oxygenated blood returning from the lungs to the left atrium is shunted back to the right atrium where it is again returned to the lungs, displacing deoxygenated blood.

Symptoms may be few, depending upon the degree of the defect but can include:

- Asymptomatic (some infants).
- Congestive heart failure.
- Heart murmur.
- Increased risk for dysrhythmias and pulmonary vascular obstructive disease over time

Treatment may not be necessary for small defects, but larger defects require closure:

- Open-heart surgical repair may be done.
- Heart catheterization and placing of closure device (Amplatz® device) across the atrial septal defect.

Hypoplastic Left Heart Syndrome (HLHS)

Hypoplastic left heart syndrome (HLHS) is underdevelopment of the left ventricle and ascending aortic atresia causing inability of the heart to pump blood, so most blood flows from the left atrium through the foramen ovale to the right atrium and to the lungs with the descending aorta receiving blood through the ductus arteriosus. There may be valvular abnormalities as well. Symptoms may be mild until the ductus arteriosus closes at about 2 weeks causing a marked increase in cyanosis and decreased cardiac output.

Symptoms include:

- Increasing cyanosis.
- Decreased cardiac output leading to cardiovascular collapse.

Mortality rates are 100% without surgical correction and 25% with correction. *Surgical procedures* include a series of 3 staged operations:

- Norwood procedure connects the main pulmonary artery to the aorta, a shunt for pulmonary blood flow, and creates a large atrial septal defect.
- Glenn procedure.
- Fontan repair procedure.
- Heart transplantation in infancy is preferred in many cases, but the shortage of hearts limits this option.

Aortic Stenosis

Aortic stenosis is a stricture (narrowing) of the aortic valve that controls the flow of blood from the left ventricle, causing the left ventricular wall to thicken as it increases pressure to overcome the valvular resistance, increasing afterload, and increasing the need for blood supply from the coronary arteries. This condition may result from a birth defect or childhood rheumatic fever and tends to worsen as over the years as the heart grows.

Symptoms include:

- Chest pain on exertion and intolerance of exercise.
- Heart murmur.
- Hypotension on exertion may be associated with sudden fainting.
- Sudden death can occur.
- Tachycardia with faint pulse.

- Poor feeding.
- Increased risk for bacterial endocarditis and coronary insufficiency.
- Increases mitral regurgitation and secondary pulmonary hypertension.

Treatment in children may be done before symptoms develop because of the danger of sudden death. Treatment includes:

- Balloon valvuloplasty to dilate valve non-surgically.
- Surgical repair of valve or replacement of valve, depending upon the extent of stricture.

Atrioventricular (AV) Canal Defect

Atrioventricular canal defect (endocardial cushion defect) is often associated with Down syndrome and involves a number of different defects, including openings between the atria and ventricles as well as abnormalities of the valves. In partial defects, there is an opening between the atria and mitral valve regurgitation. In complete defects, there is a large central hole in the heart and only one common valve between the atria and ventricles. The blood may flow freely about the heart, usually from left to right. Extra blood flow to the lungs causes enlargement of the heart. Partial defects may go undiagnosed for 20 years.

Symptoms include:

- Typical congestive heart failure signs:
    o   Weakness and fatigue.
    o   Cough and/or wheezing w/ production of white or bloody sputum.
    o   Peripheral edema and ascites.
    o   Dysrhythmia and tachycardia.
- Dyspnea.
- Poor appetite.
- Failure to thrive, low weight.
- Cyanosis of skin and lips.

Treatment includes: Open-heart surgery to patch holes in the septum and valve repair or replacement.

Congestive Heart Failure

Congestive heart failure results from the inability of the heart to adequately pump the blood the body needs. In infants, it is usually secondary to cardiac abnormalities with resultant increased blood volume and blood pressure:

- ***Right-sided failure*** occurs if the right ventricle cannot effectively contract to pump blood into the pulmonary artery, causing pressure to build in the right atrium and the venous circulation. This venous hypertension causes generalized edema of lower extremities, distended abdomen from ascites, hepatomegaly and jugular venous distension.
- ***Left-sided failure*** occurs if the left ventricle cannot effectively pump blood into the aorta and systemic circulation, increasing pressure in the left atrium and the pulmonary veins, with resultant pulmonary edema and increased pulmonary pressure. Symptoms include respiratory distress with tachypnea, grunting respirations, sternal retraction, and rales, failure to thrive and difficulty eating, often leaving the child exhausted and sweaty.

Children often have some combination of right and left-sided failure. Increased pressure in the lungs after birth may delay symptoms for 1-2 weeks.

Management of congestive heart failure (CHF) in infants can be difficult. It is extremely important to establish the etiology and to treat the underlying cause. For infants with structural cardiac abnormalities, surgical repair may be needed to resolve the CHF. There are some medical treatments that can relieve symptoms:

- *Diuretics,* such as furosemide (Lasix®), metolazone, or hydrochlorothiazide to reduce pulmonary and peripheral edema.
- *Antihypertensives*, such as Captopril® or Propranolol® to decrease heart workload.
- *Cardiac glycosides*, such as Lanoxin®, may relieve symptoms if above medicines are not successful.
- *High caloric feedings,* either by bottle or nasogastric feeding to provide sufficient nutrients.
- *Oxygen* may be useful for some children with weak hearts.
- *Restriction of activities* to reduce stress on the heart.
- *Dopamine or dobutamine* may be given to increase the contractibility of the heart.

Hypertension

Hypertension is a relatively rare finding in the neonate. Hypertension is a systolic or mean arterial blood pressure measurement greater than the 95th percentile for the infant's birth weight, gestational age, and post-natal age. Blood pressure increases as the neonate grows and matures. Signs of elevated blood pressure include lethargy, increased apnea episodes, seizures, irritability, tachypnea, and intracranial hemorrhage. Most *causes* of hypertension in the neonate are renal in origin and include:

- Thrombus formation in the kidneys from an umbilical artery catheter (the most common cause in the NICU).
- Other vascular causes, such as renal vein thrombosis, or renal artery stenosis, or coarctation of the aorta.
- Compression of renal artery by a mass.

Non-renal causes include:

- Iatrogenesis, due to administration of dopamine, Aminophylline, or glucocorticoids.
- Neurological, secondary to seizures or intraventricular hemorrhage.
- Endocrine, secondary to congenital adrenal hyperplasia or hyperthyroidism.
- Pulmonary, secondary to pneumothorax or bronchopulmonary dysplasia.
- Medications include propanolol, hydralazine, captopril, enalapril, diazoxide, and sodium nitroprusside.

Hypotension

Hypotension is a systemic mean arterial blood pressure <2 standard deviations less that average values for gestational age. The lowest reading that is within normal limits for preterm infants are is calculated as gestational age plus five. Thus, a 31-week preterm acceptable low BP would be 31-36 mm Hg. Hypotension in the neonate most often relates to dysregulation of peripheral vascular tone and/or myocardial dysfunction. Hypotension may also occur as the result of hypocalcemia, hypovolemic, cardiogenic, or distributive shock, so determining the cause of hypotension is critical to planning appropriate intervention. Early signs of hypotension are those of compensated shock and later signs of decompensated shock. Tachycardia, respiratory distress, pallor, lethargy, and cyanosis may be evident. Dopamine (2-20 μg/kg/min) is the most commonly used drug to treat neonatal hypotension as it improves myocardial function and improves peripheral vascular tension without causing vasodilation. Oxygen is administered to combat hypoxia as well as saline bolus (10-20 mL/kg).

Shock

Shock is the result of circulatory failure in which there is inadequate perfusion to meet the metabolic needs of the body. There are a number of different causes, but the physiologic responses are essentially the same:

- Hypotension (which may not be present initially because of reactive vasoconstriction).
- Hypoxemia resulting in hypoxic tissue.
- Metabolic acidosis.

There are essentially 3 stages in the progression of the shock response:

- *Compensated shock:* The sympathetic nervous response causes vasoconstriction, which may mask essential underlying hypotension but serves to provide blood flow for vital organ functions although there may be decreased circulation at the microvascular (small vessel) level.
- *Uncompensated shock:* the cardiovascular system is unable to adequately compensate and microvascular perfusion decreases.
- *Irreversible/terminal shock:* Damage to internal organs, such as the heart and brain, is so extensive that therapeutic measures cannot reverse eventual death.

Compensated Shock

During **compensated shock**, the blood pressure may remain normal initially as the compensatory sympathetic nervous response results in vasoconstriction and an increase in the heart rate and contractibility that combine to maintain cardiac output at a level adequate to supply the heart and brain while shifting circulation from other organs:

- The skin: This causes the skin to be cold and clammy.
- Gastrointestinal tract: Bowel sounds may be absent or decreased.
- Kidneys: Urinary output decreases.

Because of a decrease is tissue perfusion; lactic acid begins to build up, producing metabolic acidosis. The acidosis results in an increased respiratory rate, which serves to expel excess carbon dioxide. However, this also raises the pH of the blood and may result in respiratory alkalosis. Fluid replacement and medications to increase blood pressure and perfusion of the tissues are critical during this stage.

Decompensated Shock

Decompensated shock occurs as the body can no longer compensate, the blood pressure falls below normal, and all organs systems suffer from hypoperfusion. The heart is overworked and becomes dysfunctional and chemical changes cause myocardial depression, so that the heart begins to fail. The permeability of the capillaries increases with fluid buildup in the interstitial tissues and decreased venous return to the heart. Multi-system effects occur:

- **_Respiratory_**: respirations become rapid and shallow as the hypoxemia causes an inflammatory response and pulmonary edema, with collapse of alveoli and fibrotic changes in the lung tissue.
- **_Cardiovascular_**: Dysrhythmias and ischemia of the myocardium result in tachycardia. The myocardium is depressed and ventricles may dilate.
- **_Neurological_**: Hypoperfusion of the brain leads to changes in mental status, including lethargy and loss of consciousness. Pupils may dilate or react sluggishly.
- **_Renal_**: Acute renal failure occurs with decrease in urinary output, increase in BUN and creatinine, and electrolyte shifts.
- **_Hepatic_**: The liver loses the ability to filter and metabolize medications and metabolic waste products. Liver enzymes rise, and the skin becomes jaundiced.
- **_Gastrointestinal_**: Mucosal ulcerations may occur, causing bleeding and bloody diarrhea. Bacterial toxins may invade the lymphatic system where they are carried to the bloodstream, causing infection and increasing adverse cardiovascular responses.
- **_Hematologic_**: Disseminated vascular coagulation (DIC) may occur with both clotting and bleeding. The skin may show ecchymoses and petechiae. Clotting times are prolonged.

Treatment during this stage is dependent upon the underlying cause but includes intravenous fluids, medications to control blood pressure, cardiac function, infection, and gastrointestinal ulcerations and bleeding. Ventilatory support with oxygen and administration of sodium bicarbonate may be needed to treat metabolic acidosis. The infant must be monitored constantly, including hemodynamic monitoring, blood gases, urinary function, EKG, fluid and electrolytes, blood chemistries, enzyme levels, and neurological status.

Irreversible/Terminal Shock

The **irreversible/terminal stage of shock** can be difficult to determine because the progression of shock is a continuum rather than clearly defined stages, so the usual strategy is to continue to treat the patient with fluids, vasoactive medications to improve cardiac function, and nutritional support. During this stage hypotension persists, and complete liver and renal failure occurs. As perfusion causes necrosis of tissue, the toxins created result in severe metabolic acidosis. There is also increased lactic acidosis. Adenosine triphosphate (ATP) levels are depleted and there are no mechanisms left to store energy. Multiple organ dysfunction syndrome (MODS) occurs. There is no specific treatment that can reverse MODS, so treatment at this point becomes supportive. The mortality rate for MODS ranges from 30-100%, depending upon the number of organ systems that are involved.

Cardiogenic Shock

Cardiogenic shock in infants usually relates to congenital heart disease (usually with systemic to pulmonary shunting), myocarditis, and dysrhythmias, such as AV block and paroxysmal atrial tachycardia. These disorders interfere with the pumping mechanism of the heart, decreasing oxygen perfusion. Cardiogenic shock has 3 characteristics:

- Increased preload.
- Increased afterload.
- Decreased contractibility.

Together these result in a decreased cardiac output and an increase in systemic vascular resistance (SVR) to compensate and protect vital organs. This results in an increase of afterload in the left ventricle with increased need for oxygen. As the cardiac output continues to decrease, tissue perfusion decreases, coronary artery perfusion decreases, fluid backs up and the left ventricle fails to adequately pump the blood, resulting in pulmonary edema and right ventricular failure.

Normal Cardiac Rates

Normal cardiac rates can vary widely from one infant to another, so it's important to understand the normal range in order to determine if the infant has an abnormal pulse. Rates will also vary depending upon whether the infant is awake, sleeping, or active. Pulse rate should be taken with a stethoscope because the pulse may be difficult to palpate or count accurately manually. Additionally, this allows assessment for heart murmurs.

- Newborn infant:
    o At rest: 100-180
    o Asleep: 80-160
    o Active/sick: ≤ 220
- 1-12 weeks:
    o At rest: 100-220
    o Asleep: 80-200
    o Active/sick: ≤ 220

Monitoring of heart rate is particularly important as alterations of heart rate occur with periods of apnea. A period of apnea is usually followed by decreased heart rate as well as decrease in oxygen saturation. Respiratory rates should be monitored as well as heart rate.

Cardiac Dysrhythmias

Cardiac **dysrhythmias**, abnormal heart beats, although more common in adults can occur and are frequently the result of damage to the conduction system during major cardiac surgery.

Bradydysrhythmias are pulse rates that are abnormally slow:

- *Complete atrioventricular block (A-V block)* may be congenital or a response to surgical trauma.
- *Sinus bradycardia* may be caused by the autonomic nervous system or a response to hypotension and decrease in oxygenation.
- *Junctional/nodal rhythms* often occur in post-surgical patients when absence of P wave is noted but heart rate and output usually remain stable, and unless there is compromise, usually no treatment is necessary.

Tachydysrhythmias are pulse rates that are abnormally fast:

- *Sinus tachycardia* is often caused by illness, such as fever or infection.
- *Supraventricular tachycardia* (200-300 bpm) may have a sudden onset and result in congestive heart failure.

Conduction irregularities are irregular pulses that often occur post-operatively and are usually not significant:

- *Premature contractions* may arise from the atria or ventricles.

Cardioversion Procedure for Each Relevant Arrythmia Type

Arrhythmia Type/Cardioversion Procedure

- **Stable tachyarrhythmia:** Vagal maneuver to increase parasympathetic input to the heart and slow it. Apply ice to the neonate's face, which triggers the diving response to slow the heart rate. If unsuccessful, try adenosine, digoxin, or propanolol.
- **Unstable arrhythmia with narrow QRS complex:** Synchronized electrical cardioversion is appropriate for atrial flutter or fibrillation, WPW, or PJRT. Set the defibrillator for 0.5 to 2.0 Joules/kg. Place two electrode pads on the infant's chest. Wait for the optimum moment in the cardiac cycle. Pass electrical current through the infant's heart.
- **Unstable arrhythmia with wide QRS complex:** Asynchronous cardioversion is appropriate for ventricular tachycardia or fibrillation, SVT with BBB, or antidromic SVT in WPW. Defibrillate because there is no R wave present to time the shock.
- **Stable arrhythmia with wide QRS complex:** Try esophageal pacing. If unresponsive, try procainamide and lidocaine. Follow with Flecainide if unresponsive. Asynchronous cardioversion at 2 j/kg, 2 j/kg, and 4j/kg, if necessary.
- **Bradyarrhythmias:** For 1:1 sinus bradycardia, complete AV block, Wenckebach's phenomenon, and sinus exit block: Check airway, breathing, and circulation. Treat underlying cause. Give oxygen, atropine, and isoproterenol. Start transvenous pacing.

Pulmonary

Respiratory Distress Syndrome

Respiratory distress syndrome (RDS) (hyaline membrane disease) occurs in 14% of low birth weight infants. RDS is caused by the absence or deficiency of surfactant. Surfactant is a lipoprotein that reduces surface tension in the alveoli. Surfactant causes the lungs to be more compliant (alveoli expand with less effort) and the alveoli do not collapse on end expiration. Surfactant production begins at 22 weeks of gestation, but levels are inadequate until 36 weeks of gestation. Lack of surfactant produces alveolar collapse (atelectasis) and less compliant lungs that cause laborious breathing. Collapsed areas of lung may still receive blood flow, but no exchange of gases occurs (ventilation perfusion mismatch). If RDS is left untreated, hypoxemia and hypercarbia develop, leading to respiratory acidosis. Acidosis and hypoxemia lead to a cycle of increased pulmonary vascular resistance and vasoconstriction, causing increased hypoxemia.

Air Leak Syndrome

Premature infants have fragile lung tissue and often require positive pressure ventilation (PPV), ventilator support, and administration of pulmonary drugs (e.g., surfactant), making them susceptible to **air leak syndrome**. As pressure increases inside alveoli, the alveolar wall pulls away from the perivascular sheath and subsequent alveolar rupture allows air to follow the perivascular planes and flow into adjacent areas. There are numerous types of air leaks:

- Pneumothorax (spontaneous or traumatic) is air in the pleural space.
- Tension pneumothorax is one-way airflow into the pleural cavity, with pressure build-up and significant collapse of lung tissue, causing respiratory compromise.
- Pneumoperitoneum is air in the peritoneal area, including the abdomen and occasionally the scrotal sac of male infants.
- Pneumomediastinum is air in the mediastinal area between the lungs.
- Pneumopericardium is air in the pericardial sac that surrounds the heart.
- Subcutaneous emphysema is air in the subcutaneous tissue planes of the chest wall.
- Pulmonary interstitial emphysema (PIE) is air trapped in the interstitium between the alveoli.

Pneumothorax

Pneumothorax is the most common type of air leak syndrome. In infants, increased air pressure caused by the use of mechanical ventilation is the most common cause, but infants may develop spontaneous pneumothorax, especially those infants with fragile lung tissue are at high risk:

- Infants with lung disease, including hyaline membrane disease (HMD).
- Premature infants.
- Infants with meconium aspiration.

Symptoms vary according to the type of pneumothorax (spontaneous, traumatic, or tension) but can include:

- ↑Respiratory distress with tachypnea and chest wall retractions
- Absence of breath sounds on auscultation.
- Paradoxical chest movement in which the chest contracts during inhalation and expands during exhalation.
- Shift in maximum intensity sounds of heart.
- Bradycardia and cyanosis.

Treatment includes:

- Evacuating air with needle aspiration or chest tubes to water seal drainage.
- Correction of underlying cause.

Apnea of Prematurity

Premature infants (especially those <34 weeks) often exhibit **apnea of prematurity (AOP).** AOP begins at birth and is believed caused by immaturity of the nervous system, improving as the brain matures. It may persist for a 4-8 weeks. There are 3 types of apnea:

- Central: no airflow or effort to breathe.
- Obstructive: no airflow, but effort to breathe.
- Mixed: both central and obstructive elements (75% of AOP).

AOP *symptoms* include:

- Swallowing during apneic periods.
- Apnea >20 seconds.
- Apnea < 20 seconds with bradycardia 30 beats <normal.
- Oxygen saturation <85% persisting ≥5 seconds.
- Cyanosis.

Treatment includes:

- Tactile stimulation (rubbing limbs or thorax or gently slapping bottoms of feet) or gently lifting the jaw to relieve obstruction.
- Oxygen or bag/mask ventilation for bradycardia and ↓oxygen saturation. Continuous positive airway pressure (CPAP) for mixed or obstructive apnea. Aminophylline/theophylline or caffeine (for central apnea) may increase contractions of diaphragm.

Meconium Aspiration Syndrome

Meconium aspiration syndrome (MAS) occurs when meconium, expelled in the amniotic fluid (occurring in about 20% of pregnancies), is aspirated by the fetus *in utero* or the neonate at first breath. Blood and amniotic fluids may be aspirated as well. Some infants may present with *symptoms* at birth, but sometimes symptoms are delayed for a number of hours:

- Tachypnea.
- Lethargy, depressed state.
- Hypoxemia and hypercapnia.
- Metabolic acidosis may occur.
- Hyperventilation may occur in early stages with hypoventilation in later stages.

Symptoms are similar to transient tachypnea of the newborn (TTN) but they are more severe and the infant appears more compromised. Chest x-rays may show infiltrates, atelectasis, hypoinflated areas as well as hyperinflated areas. Pulmonary hypertension may result. *Treatment* includes:

- Preventive suctioning of the oropharynx as soon as the head is delivered.
- Intubation and suctioning of the trachea for infants with respiratory distress (weak respirations, bradycardia, hypotonia).
- Supplemental oxygen and/or mechanical ventilation as indicated.

Persistent Pulmonary Hypertension

Persistent pulmonary hypertension (PPHN) occurs when the high pulmonary vascular pressure that keeps fetal blood from circulating through the lungs fails to reduce after birth, so that blood continues to bypass the lungs, and the foramen ovale and ductus arteriosus are forced by pressure to remain open with venous blood shunting into systemic circulation instead of being oxygenated in the lungs. Infants are usually near or full-term, but present at birth with respiratory distress and cyanosis. PPHN is the cause of about 50% of neonatal deaths. There are 3 classifications:

- **Primary** is idiopathic with normal lung tissue but arterial hyperplasia and/or premature constricting of ductus arteriosus *in utero.*
- **Secondary** is precipitated by another disorder, such as meconium aspiration pneumonia (MAP), transient tachypnea of the newborn (TTN) or hyaline membrane disease. This is the most common form.
- **Hypoplastic** is related to pulmonary hypoplasia with anatomic changes in alveoli and vasculature in the lung.

PPHN has been linked to maternal use of SSRIs and NSAIDs.

Symptoms are usually evident within the first 12 hours of birth and progress over the next 24-48 hours:

- Cyanosis with poor cardiac perfusion, tachycardia. Hypoxemia, persisting even with supplemental oxygen.
- Systolic murmur with regurgitation of the tricuspid valve.
- Tachypnea and general respiratory distress.

Treatment for **persistent pulmonary hypertension (PPHN)** will be specific for the underlying cause, and can include:

- Intubation and mechanical ventilation with HFV especially with parenchymal lung disease.
- Central venous lines for administration of solutions, such as calcium gluconate.
- Arterial line to monitor arterial blood gas.
- Surfactants (beractant) to reduce surface tension in patients without primary PPHN.
- High frequency ventilation (HFV) is used with underlying lung disease resulting in low volume.
- Extracorporeal membrane oxygenation (ECMO) is used if other forms of support are not successful, and most often if the infant also has congenital diaphragmatic hernia.
- Sodium bicarbonate is often used to correct metabolic acidosis in practice, however there is no evidence of short or long-term benefits.
- Sedation (fentanyl) to reduce restlessness. Induced paralysis (pancuronium, vecuronium) has been used but is implicated in increased mortality rates, atelectasis, sensory hearing loss, and ventilation-perfusion mismatch.
- Inhaled nitrous oxide.

Pneumonia

Type of infection / Causes / Pathogens

Transplacental infection / Aspiration of infected amniotic fluid. The pathogen crosses the placenta directly from the mother. / Cytomegalovirus, rubella, *Toxoplasmosis gondii*, varicella and *Listeria monocytogenes*

Intrapartal infection / Intrauterine infection when membranes have been ruptured for a prolonged time. Infant contracts the pathogen during passage through the birthing canal. / Herpes simplex virus, chlamydia, Group B *Streptococci*, *Klebsiella* and *Escherichia coli*

Post-partal infection / Nosocomial (hospital-acquired) infection / *Staphylococcus aureus, S. epidermidis,* herpes simplex, *Candida albicans*, cytomegalovirus, Group B *Streptococci*, and respiratory syncytial virus.

Hospital-Acquired Pneumonias

Klebsiella pneumoniae is a common cause of hospital-acquired infections of the urinary tract, surgical sites, and lower respiratory tract. *K. Pneumoniae* is a Gram-negative member of the Enterobacteriaceae family and is part of the normal body flora. It can infect children of all ages but is most common in infants who are premature and/or in neonatal intensive care. Infants with invasive devices, such as those with mechanical ventilation, are at increased risk. There have been a number of outbreaks in neonatal units, especially with multi-drugs resistant forms, with the hands of health staff and the gastrointestinal tract of the infants providing reservoirs of bacteria. When the infection attacks the lungs, the *symptoms* include inflammatory changes that result in necrosis and hemorrhage, clogging the lungs with thick puro-sanguinous exudate. The disease spreads rapidly, with high fever and dyspnea. Mortality rates are high. *Treatment* includes antibiotic therapy (such as 3rd generation cephalosporins or quinolones) based on cultures and sensitivities.

Hospital-acquired pneumonias (HAP) are far more lethal than community-acquired pneumonias (CAP), with HAP death rates of 20-40% and up to 90% if the infant is on mechanical ventilation, with *Pseudomonas aeruginosa* one of the most lethal (40-60% mortality) because it can invade blood vessels, resulting in hemorrhage. Most infections are spread by contact with contaminated hands of healthcare staff or from invasive devices, such as endotracheal tubes, and mechanical ventilators. *Symptoms* include fever, cough, bradycardia, and elevated WBC counts.

Treatment includes:

- Antibiotic therapy: Usually combinations of 2 antibiotics are given, such as piperacillin or ceftazidime AND gentamicin or ciprofloxacin (based on cultures). Vancomycin is generally avoided because of the rise of vancomycin-resistant organisms.
- Preventive measures include maintaining ventilated patients in 30° upright positions, universal precautions, and changing ventilator circuits as per protocol.

Pulmonary Hemorrhage

Pulmonary hemorrhage is bleeding within the alveoli. This usually is the result of some other event, such as intracranial hemorrhage, asphyxia, aspiration, heart disease, or sepsis. This can also be the result of a trauma from over-aggressive suctioning. Pulmonary hemorrhage presents as bright red blood from the trachea found with suctioning and as rapid, sudden respiratory deterioration. Pulmonary hemorrhage can cause rapid death if the bleeding is severe and is often only found during an autopsy. A more minor hemorrhage can be managed with blood transfusions and assisted ventilation. Pulmonary hemorrhage may result in hemothorax. In some cases, pneumothorax may also be present, resulting in mediastinal shift that increases the difficulty of identifying and repairing the bleeding vessel. If the infant is stabilized, computed tomography may provide accurate diagnosis to isolate the area of hemorrhage. The underlying cause of the hemorrhage must be discovered and treated.

Pulmonary hemorrhage is sometimes treated with surfactant although there are no adequate randomized studies at this time to show efficacy. However, preliminary reports appear positive. In some cases, pulmonary hemorrhage may be associated with the use of surfactant. The use of surfactant therapy is common in preterm infants to reduce morbidity and mortality related to respiratory distress syndrome. It is also sometimes used for infants receiving prolonged ventilatory support. Surfactant improves lung compliance, decreases pulmonary vascular resistance, and increases flow (right to left) through a patent ductus arteriosus or persistent foramen ovale. However, these very improvements in lung function can result in pulmonary hemorrhage, especially in ventilatory support is not adjusted with respect to the improved pulmonary function, so it's very important that ventilation be monitored carefully after administration of surfactant.

Pulmonary Hypoplasia

Pulmonary hypoplasia occurs when the lungs and component parts are present but severely underdeveloped with less volume, decreased alveoli, fewer airway generations, and decreased pulmonary arteries. Pulmonary hypoplasia may result from congenital diaphragmatic hernia or embryologic defect that may include various other anomalies, such as prune-belly or Potter syndrome. Fetal urine in the amniotic fluid is necessary for development of fetal lungs, so renal agenesis or obstruction results in pulmonary hypoplasia. Hypoplasia is usually a secondary rather than primary disorder. If the hypoplasia is the result of compression caused by a diaphragmatic hernia, then after surgical repair, the lung will partially recover. Mortality rates range from 70-95%, depending upon severity and other anomalies. Preventive methods include providing amnio-infusions for preterm ruptured membranes <32 weeks to reduce hypoplasia. After birth, treatment includes:

- Respiratory support: supplemental oxygen or ventilation (HFOV and EMCO).
- Surfactants (Survanta®) to improve ventilation and oxygenation.
- Surgical repair as indicated.
- Vasodilators and/or bronchial dilators as indicated.

Congenital Diaphragmatic Hernia

Congenital diaphragmatic hernias (CDH) may cause severe respiratory distress. The primary CDHs that affect infants are posterolateral (Bochdalek):

- Left sided (85%) includes herniation of the large and small intestine and intraabdominal organs into the thoracic cavity.
- Right sided (13%) may be asymptomatic or involve usually just the liver and part of the large intestine herniate.

Neonates with left CDH may exhibit severe respiratory distress and cyanosis. The lungs may be underdeveloped because of pressure exerted from displaced organs during fetal development. There may be a left hemothorax with a mediastinal shift and the heart pressing on the right lung, which may be hypoplastic. Bowel sounds are heard over the chest area. Pulmonary hypertension and cardiopulmonary failure may occur. Treatment includes:

- Surgical repair after stabilization
- HFOV for pulmonary hypoplasia.
- Extracorporeal membrane oxygenation (ECMO) for cardiopulmonary dysfunction.

Nitric oxide is a controversial but frequently used treatment. It doesn't decrease mortality but does help quickly stabilize patients and reduce the incident of arrest. Despite treatment, mortality rates are 50%, and children who survive may have emphysema, with larger volume but inadequate numbers of alveoli.

Bronchopulmonary Dysplasia

Bronchopulmonary dysplasia (BFD) is a chronic lung disease characterized by alveolar damage resulting from abnormal development with inflammation and development of scar tissue. Risk factors include:

- Prematurity of >10 weeks prior to due date.
- Birthweight <2.5 lbs/1000 grams.
- Hyaline membrane disease or respiratory distress syndrome (RDS) at birth.
- Long-term ventilatory support/oxygen.

Most of the infants have immature lungs with inadequate surfactant to allow the lungs to expand properly, so they cannot breathe without assistance. *Symptoms* include severe respiratory distress and cyanosis. *Treatment* includes surfactant and ventilators or nasal continuous positive airway pressure (NCPAP) to provide oxygenation and protect vital organs. Usually infants improve within 2-4 weeks, but some progress from RDS to BFD. Their lungs often have fewer but enlarged alveoli with inadequate blood supply. BFD is usually diagnosed if respiratory symptoms do not improve after 28 days.

Treatment is supportive to allow the lungs to mature:

- Mechanical ventilation or High-frequency jet ventilation (HFJV).
- Supplemental oxygen.
- Bronchodilators (albuterol) to open airways.
- Furosemide (Lasix®) to reduce pulmonary edema.
- Antibiotics as indicated.
- Gastric feedings or total parenteral nutrition (TPN)

Most infants are hospitalized for about 4 months but may need treatment for months or years at home. Most will eventually develop nearly normal lung function as new lung tissue grows and takes over the function of the scarred tissue. Some long-term complications may occur:

- Increased risk of bacterial and viral infections, such as RSV and pneumonia.
- Chronic or recurrent pulmonary edema.
- Pulmonary hypertension.
- Side effects related to long-term use of diuretics, such as hearing deficits, renal calculi, and electrolyte imbalances.
- Slow growth patterns.

Laryngomalacia and Tracheomalacia

Laryngomalacia results from a congenital shortening of the aryepiglottic folds that open and close the vocal cords. This shortening causes an omega-shaped curling of the epiglottis that causes respiratory obstruction, characterized by inspiratory strider, usually not associated with other symptoms. Strider may be absent at birth but increase over the first few weeks. This condition usually resolves by 2 years, but may, in severe cases require surgical repair.

Tracheomalacia is a congenital abnormality of the trachea in which the supporting cartilage is weak and posterior membranous wall is widened. The distal third of the trachea is most commonly affected, and the condition may be associated with other congenital defects, such as cardiovascular abnormalities. Tracheomalacia may be associated with tracheoesophageal fistula. Symptoms include expiratory stridor, cough (especially during feeding), recurrent respiratory infections, and reflex periods of apnea. Treatment includes humidified air, antibiotics, and care in feeding. This condition usually resolves as the infant grows, but in rare cases, surgery may be indicated.

Pulmonic Stenosis

Pulmonic stenosis is a stricture of the pulmonic valve that controls the flow of blood from the right ventricle to the lungs, resulting in right ventricular hypertrophy as the pressure increases in the right ventricle and decreased pulmonary blood flow. The condition may be asymptomatic or symptoms may not be evident until the child enters adulthood, depending upon the severity of the defect. Pulmonic stenosis may be associated with a number of other heart defects.

Symptoms of pulmonic stenosis can include:

- Loud heart murmur
- Congestive heart murmur
- Mild cyanosis
- Cardiomegaly
- Angina
- Dyspnea
- Fainting
- Increased risk of bacterial endocarditis

Treatment includes:

- Balloon valvuloplasty to separate the cusps of the valve for children.
- Surgical repair includes the (closed) transventricular valvotomy (Brock) procedure for infants and the cardiopulmonary bypass pulmonary valvotomy for older children